Fitness Tips

Fitness Tips

A Practical And Biblically Based Guide To Living A Healthy Life

Karen Roberts

This book is dedicated to my husband, James Roberts, for always believing in me, supporting my dreams, and being my rock. And to my children, Joshua, Justin, Andrew, and Jaron, may you all obtain great health benefits from the information in this book. Pass it on to your wives, children, and grandchildren.

Disclaimer

I am not a doctor. I have various health, wellness, and teaching certifications. Please consult your doctor or medical provider before starting any exercise and nutritional program. This information is for informational purposes only and is not intended to be a substitute for professional medical advice, practices, or use. I encourage you, as I do my clients, to not just take my advice, but do your own research to determine the right program for you.

Finally, some of the information used in this book is my opinion, based on my educational background, unless otherwise noted.

Thank you.

Table of Contents

Foreword

I was honored to be asked by my wife, Karen Roberts, to write an acknowledgment for her book. She is a Certified Personal Trainer, Certified Food Over Medicine Instructor, and Certified Nutrition Coach, and working with her in our personal coaching business lets me know you are in for a treat if you want to improve your health. I watched her study and assemble all this information so that the reader would get the best of knowledge, wisdom, and ease of understanding.

Karen has helped numerous amounts of people reach their goals through using physical activity and healthy nutrition. She works tirelessly. She is more than qualified to give you the coaching you need to improve your health outcomes. The word of God says in Jeremiah 29:11 New Living Translation, *"For I know the plans I have for you," "They are plans for good and not for disaster, to give you a future and hope."* Karen understands that with the knowledge of living a lifestyle of meaningful, healthy choices, you can fulfill God's plan for good and not for disaster, to give you a future of great health and hope for your families.

Plus, the information in this book is biblically based because, without the help of the Holy Spirit, we could do nothing. I know this book will open your eyes to what it could be if you apply it to your life. She not only has information that is scientifically based, but also full of informative information that will lead you to good health, spiritually, physically, and mentally, as well as enlighten you to a great new life!

James Roberts, CPT, CHHNC, CNC, CWC

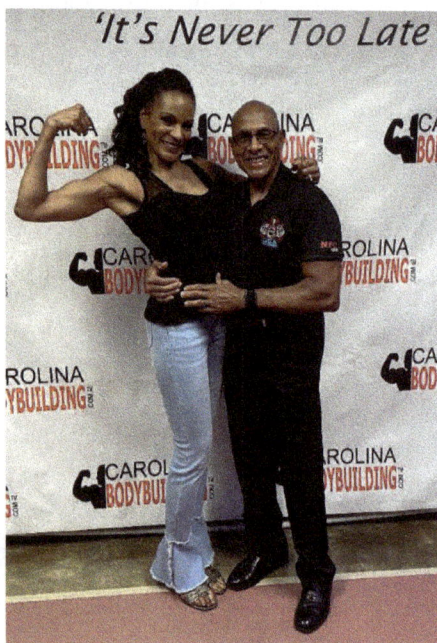

Introduction

This could be the most important book you'll ever read. It contains invaluable fitness tips that could guide you to a healthier lifestyle. I was inspired to write this book due to training my clients, sharing my knowledge on the radio, and constantly answering fitness-related questions. I am a Christian, and I believe the Bible, along with the Holy Spirit, leads us in the direction that God would have us to go in. So, there will be bible verses as we read to remind us of God's will for our lives.

People tend to think that health and wellness is all about our bodies from the neck down. Our heart, lungs, body weight, fat/lean percentage, and so on. And all of that is true.

However, that is only part of the story. We also have a neck-up. Our mindset has a lot to do with our physical health. That's why I opened this book with a mental component. You can have the most physically fit body in the world, but without the mental fortitude, it's almost impossible to get through workouts or even make the simplest healthy food choices. As humans, we experience a wide range of emotions, from elation to depression, depending on what may be going on in our lives. The food we eat, and whether or not we work out, will have a direct impact on our mental well-being and how we handle our emotions. Not only that, but it may also determine whether or not we get mental diseases that affect our brains, such as dementia.

So it is vitally important that we focus on our health from head to toe.

Chapter Two points out the metabolic challenges we could experience based on our food choices. Metabolic disease occurs when an abnormal chemical reaction in the body disturbs the normal process of achieving energy. Food is broken down by the body into a chemical form, which is then distributed throughout the body to provide energy. Unhealthy food choices may have an adverse effect on the body. Too much or too little of certain nutrients in the body can lead to metabolic diseases, such as type II diabetes, obesity, arthritis, high cholesterol or Blood Pressure, and more. Knowing which foods to eat and avoid, may help in staffing off these diseases.

Chapter Three tackles the body and movement. The saying, "Move it or lose it," is not just a slogan, but a reality. There is nothing we can do to stop Mother Nature and the aging of our bodies. However, adverse genes aside, we can slow down the process. If we don't move our bodies, as we age, we will begin to see a rapid decline in movement, strength, and flexibility. So, it is essential that we find ways to move our bodies. Not everyone is meant to go to the gym, whether the reason is financial, access/availability, or other. However, every able-bodied person should find a way to be active. The Bible says God put us here to work (Genesis 2:15). This will keep us healthy, wealthy (and I don't mean in a financial way), and wise. What good is it having all the money in the world, but not being able to enjoy it because you're sick, bedridden, and not able to move?

Chapter Four gives us a micro breakdown of tips that we can do on a daily basis. Most of us live in areas that have multiple seasons. And with that comes many challenges. Adaptations vary depending on your life, where you live, if you're married, have children, and so on. Then you may live in an area where the summers are scorching hot, or just the opposite, with brutal snow-laden winters. Having to deal with that, and a family, or pets, or whatever your circumstances are, all affect your lifestyle, the food you have access to, and the makeup of your exercise program. I pray some of these tips will give you just the boost you need to get through the day, or to make it to the next season.

Chapter Five addresses our children. Without healthy children, our future is dim, at best. Some of the tips I share here address some of the metabolic diseases plaguing our children. The tips will hopefully bring awareness to the issues, and ways to prevent, slow down, and or reverse any issues that may (potentially) exist. These issues are addressed with dietary and exercise tips that hopefully will last a lifetime.

Chapter Six is designed to make us look at our eating habits. It addresses what we may be doing vs. what we could be doing to get better health outcomes. The tips touch on certain foods, herbs, spices, and some minerals to help boost the health of our body, and thus, the quality of our life.

Finally, Chapter Seven contains recipes, including a smoothie recipe, breakfast, lunch, and dinner. As I said in the beginning, the food we eat will have a profound impact on our health, for better or worse. I felt it was important to add the nutritional value of the ingredients in each recipe so you have all the health benefits, thus making it the largest chapter in the book. It is important to know how food affects your body, thus giving you the proper tools to determine if it is a food you want to eat. Just because a food is listed as being healthy, it doesn't mean you should eat it. Strawberries are a healthy food. However, I am allergic to strawberries, so I don't eat them. Also, recipes can be customized to fit your metabolic needs and taste. So, I pray there are some recipes that fit your taste buds and that you share them with your family and friends.

I pray that these tips will help you understand your health better. I pray you will take control over what goes into your body, and live a lifestyle that will move you in the direction of being stronger, fitter, and wiser as you age.

Chapter 1 - Mental

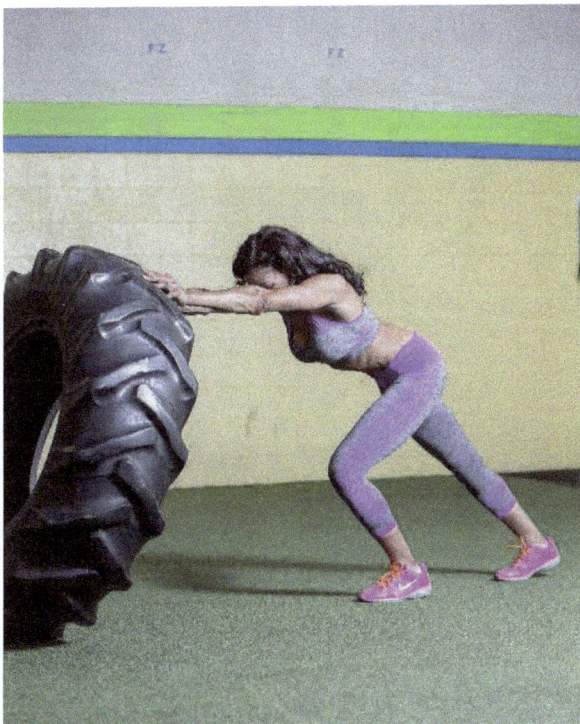

Believing in yourself is half the battle. Doing the work is the other half. When you challenge yourself, only the sky is the limit to what you can accomplish.

Upgrading Our Mindset

When it comes to eating clean and exercising, many start with good intentions, but as soon as a bump in the road comes along, or life throws us a curve, we revert to our old comfortable ways of skipping working out and eating unhealthy foods. We make excuses to justify our bad habits.

So, I want to talk about getting our MINDSET RIGHT to MAKE THE CHANGES WE NEED to live a clean and healthy life.

The Bible says:

"Do not be conformed to this world, but be transformed by the renewal of your mind, that by testing, you may discern God's will and what is good and acceptable and perfect." - Romans 12:2.

When we decide to make "major" changes in our lives, we have to start with our MINDSET. When things happen (foreseen and unforeseen), we are better prepared to tough it out!

Your mindset and belief system affect everything in your life, from what you think and feel to how you act and react to the world around you.

To achieve your goals, your mindset needs to match your aspirations. Otherwise, it might be holding you back from getting where you want to be.

So here are three steps to take to get you started:

1. Change "your self-talk" and your focus.

Here's the thing...

The things we say MANIFEST… so if You're constantly saying I'm not good enough for this or I don't think I can achieve that GOAL, those are the things that will come to fruition.

TRY TO always speak in the **affirmative**!

Change what you're saying, for example: "I know I can do this," or "If it's never been done, then I'll be the first to do it." Or… I WILL GO INTO THIS SITUATION WITH AN OPEN MIND, OR LET'S SEE WHAT HAPPENS WHEN WE SWITCH THINGS UP.

You need to be just that positive!

Also, FOCUS ON having a positive mindset, as This encourages a mentality of "abundance" instead of "fear, defeat, and lack."

2. ACT as if you've already achieved the goal:

Ever heard someone say, fake it until you make it?

We need to be obedient to what GOD tells us to do!

"You see that a person is justified by works and not by faith alone."

- James 2:24.

Having faith is great! But, The way to achieve your goal is to WORK towards it... so if your goal is to be lean, healthy, and fit:

You have to ACT like people who are lean, healthy, and fit. Do your research, read, and listen to books & magazines that help guide you to your goal!

- Talk to your doctor,
- talk to people already doing what you want to do,
- Eat clean,
- Exercise,
- Drink plenty of water... and more…

And you will see, with determination, dedication, and Commitment, you will achieve your goals in due time, and…

3. As I am known for saying, surround yourself with like-minded people:

This is one of the reasons we all go to church! As Christians, we support, fellowship, and uplift each other. This is important in all areas of our life, not just in church. It's easier to do something when everyone around is doing the same thing. In other words, it's tough to eat a salad when everyone else around you is eating pizza and burgers. On the other hand, it is very easy to eat a salad when everyone around you is eating salad.

"But be doers of the word, and not hearers only, deceiving yourselves."

- James 1:22.

You may have to make some changes in your lifestyle, but the good news is that the more conducive your environment is to your goals, the more you will likely stick to them.

So, let's not be stuck on where we are and get our mindset focused on where we want to be!

To paraphrase pastor Mike: "I look a whole lot better in the future than I do right now. And I want you too, ALSO."

I hope it's been a blessing! Please pass it on to family and friends.

Brain Health - How To Achieve And Maintain It

I want to talk to you about keeping your brain as strong and healthy as the rest of your body:

"The Lord God took the man and put him in the garden of Eden to work it and keep it."

- Genesis 2:15.

WE WERE NOT MADE TO BE IDLE, BUT TO DO THE WORK OF THE LORD, SO WE MUST STRIVE TO BE AS HEALTHY AS POSSIBLE, IN ALL AREAS, INCLUDING OUR BRAINS!

Do you know that our brain is a muscle? The same as a bicep, quad, ab, or any other muscle in the body —And our brains can atrophy(waste away) from non-use, just the same as any other muscle in the body.

Just as weight workouts add lean muscle to your body and help you retain more muscle later in your years, research shows that following a healthy lifestyle and performing regular, targeted brain exercises can also increase your brain's cognitive reserve.

In one of the most detailed studies on the connection between lifestyle and dementia risk (to date), researchers found that people who participate in *multiple healthy behaviors* significantly reduce their risk for dementia. A 2013 study published in PLOS ONE (a peer-reviewed scientific journal published by the Public Library of Science (PLOS)) looked at over 2,235 men for 30 years. It measured their participation in five healthy lifestyle behaviors:

- No Smoking,
- Optimal BMI,
- High fruit and vegetable intake,
- Regular physical activity, and
- Low to moderate alcohol intake.

The study participants who followed four or all five behaviors were about 60 percent less likely to develop cognitive impairment and dementia.

Dr. Robert Bender, medical director of the Johnny Orr Memory Center and Healthy Aging Institute in Des Moines, Iowa, says... Avoiding Ruts and Boredom is critical because... "The brain wants to learn new things," he also says; sedentary and relatively passive activities, such as sitting in front of a TV for hours a day, can be detrimental to brain health over time.

Most experts agree that even the most straightforward exercises strengthen the brain, such as:

- Driving home a different route
- Brushing your teeth with your other hand

So here is an exercise from Dr. John E. Morley, director of St. Louis University's Division of Geriatric Medicine, that you can try in your spare time.

- Test your recall.

Make a list — of grocery items, things to do, or anything else that comes to mind — and memorize it. An hour or so later, see how many items you can recall. Make items on the list as challenging as possible for the most significant mental stimulation.

And see how well you do! If you don't do well the first time, NO WORRIES... try again in a few hours/days with a different list. Watch and see how much your memory improves over time!

So now you know there are steps you can take to keep the brain just as strong and healthy as the rest of your body, and there is scientific evidence to back it up!

I pray that this message has been a blessing to you. Share this information with friends and family.

Be blessed!

Train (Memory And) Your Brain!

"Listen to advice and accept instructions, and in the end, you will be wise." (NIV)

- Proverbs 19:20.

God has given us the master plan, the information, and the tools we need to be successful... spiritually and physically...

Do you want to improve your brain? Be smarter? More alert? Then, this section is just for you.

Over the last ten years, many new medical buzzwords have taken the spotlight, like the microbiome and diabetes III being referred to as Alzheimer's, as studies show one of the probable causes is poor diet. But there is another word being used today, and that is 'Hippocampus.' This part of the brain is responsible for storing information in our memory. Studies further show that as you age, and unless you take matters into your own hands, your brain will shrink, leading to an increased risk of dementia.

So, how do we stop this from happening? Well, we have to exercise! Studies have shown that the more you exercise, the greater the blood flow to the brain (as well as throughout the

11

body), and the more the grey matter is increased, giving one more memory storage space. Unfortunately, the opposite has also been shown: the less you exercise, the more likely the brain is to shrink.

This loss typically happens (or is noticed) late in adulthood, meaning that in most cases, there is time to take preventive measures. The studies show that loss may be slowed or even reversed with exercise as training is added or increased.

This is how it works: as we exercise, the liver makes ketones (an energy source used when glucose is unavailable) from fatty acids. The ketones activate a gene that instructs the brain to enter survivor mode (BDNF- Brain Derived Neurotropic Factor) to protect itself and to ensure its longevity. The brain responds through a process called angiogenesis (growing blood vessels), which provides the pathways by which the hippocampus can sustain and maintain itself. As these new pathways are developed, it's not just long-term memory that benefits; our short-term memory also benefits.

This process improves many neuron factors, like decision-making, reaction time, mood, appetite, and diet. Now, you don't have to work out every day. Consistency is the key. In Chapter 3, I talk about exercise swaps, and throughout the book, there are varying ways to incorporate exercise as a lifestyle. So the next time you lose your keys or can't remember the details of something, think back to the last time you exercised. If it has been a while, add it to your daily regimen and see how great it feels to recall information easily again!

I pray that this message has been a blessing to you. Share this information with family and friends.

Be blessed!

Contributions made via the following article:

"Exercise training increases the size of the hippocampus and improves memory."

Kirk I Erickson 1, Michelle W Voss, Ruchika Shaurya Prakash, Chandramallika Basak, Amanda Szabo, Laura Chaddock, Jennifer S Kim, Susie Heo, Heloisa Alves, Siobhan M White, Thomas R Wojcicki, Emily Mailey, Victoria J Vieira, Stephen A Martin, Brandt D Pence, Jeffrey A Woods, Edward McAuley, Arthur F Kramer

Taking Care of Your Mental Health - Managing Negative People

"A cheerful heart is a good medicine, but a crushed spirit dries up the bones."

- Proverbs 17:22.

Negativity is a form of Toxicity.

Research shows that negativity is incredibly harmful and contagious. Happiness is something that we all strive for, especially during a pandemic. While it is nearly impossible to eliminate negative thoughts, people, and situations altogether, and although we'll always have good and bad days, we can choose to strip away the parts of our lives that bring us down and instead refocus that energy towards being the best version of ourselves.

Some of the biggest detriments to being positive come from toxic people.

We all know someone who, no matter what the situation is, always sees the glass as being half empty. These people are not fun to be around, but they can also negatively affect your health and success.

No matter how positive of a person you are, negative people can affect your life unless you take the proper precautions.

Research shows that even the smallest amount of harmful brain activity can lead to a weakened immune system, making you more prone to illness and even a heart attack and stroke.

According to Dr. Travis Bradberry, the Chief People Scientist at LEADx, a world-renowned expert in emotional intelligence, an award-winning co-author of the #1 best-selling book, *Emotional Intelligence 2.0*, and the co-founder of TalentSmart® says…

"… negativity can also affect your intelligence and ability to think by compromising the effectiveness of the neurons in the hippocampus - an important area of the brain responsible for reasoning and memory."

On top of that, negative people can:

- Affect your attitude
- Drain your energy and
- Damage your credibility

So, how do you rid yourself of unnecessary negativity and protect your mental health?

Here are three ways...

1. Say Goodbye!

Life is too short to spend around negative, crabby, grouchy people. Begin by purging the toxic people from your life and increasing the positive people in your life. You will see an increase in the quality of your life, both physically and mentally.

Seek a positive person to meet with regularly, such as for a quick lunch. This could boost your mood for the rest of the day.

2. Set Limits!

Understandably, there are people in our lives that we cannot eliminate, such as a boss or co-workers. However, you can still protect your positive attitude by setting limits and distancing yourself when possible. For example, if you encounter a person complaining about something, you can either leave the room (go back to work or another room) or ask them how they would change the situation to improve it. This puts the conversation on a positive path. And...

3. We all know that negative people are contagious, but so are positive people!

Have you ever heard of "paying it forward"? Paying it forward (PIF) means repaying a kindness received with a good deed to someone else.

Multiple studies have shown that PIF not only makes others feel better, but it creates long-lasting feelings of joy within yourself and can be an overall mood booster.

How can you do this? There are many ways, but two great ways are one, bring some healthy treats to work one day, or two, offer to help with a project.

So, if there are negative people around you (business or personal), try some strategies to reduce or eliminate the impact of toxic people in your life and your health. Your mind and body will thank you!

I pray that this message has been a blessing to you. Share this information with friends and family and share the good news that living fit offers.

Be blessed!

Marcy Welch shows in this picture what is possible when you make up your mind.

Chapter 2 – Metabolic Care

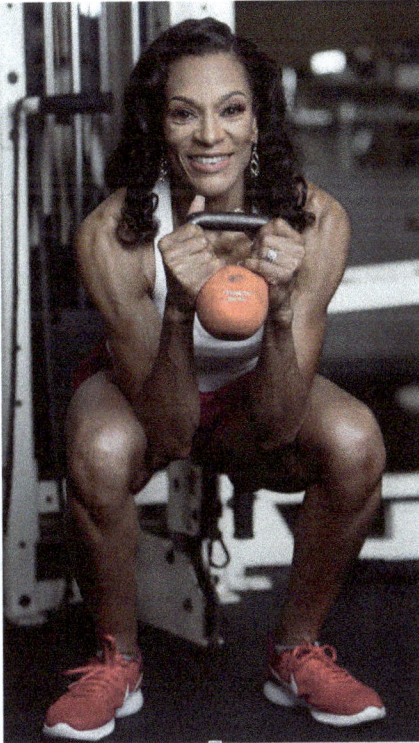

Working out does not always have to be with dumbbells or machines.

Kettlebells can rev up any workout!

Pre-Diabetes

What is pre-diabetes? Pre-diabetes can be a blessing in disguise.

"Diabetes." For some, it is an overused buzzword. The response can be pretty visceral for those managing it or working to keep it at bay.

"Pre-diabetes." A term used more frequently lately. For some, this diagnosis can be a blessing in disguise.

What is pre-diabetes?

WebMD describes it as "a wake-up call that you're on the path to diabetes, but it's not too late to turn things around." It's when blood sugar levels are higher than usual but not yet high enough to be classified as type 2 diabetes. This means a fasting glucose test in the 100-125 range or an A1C trial between 5.7 and 6.4 percent.

Without intervention or some shifts in lifestyle, pre-diabetes is likely to become diabetes.

Having pre-diabetes may mean that long-term damage to the circulatory system and heart is in progress.

According to a 2014 Centers for Disease Control and Prevention (CDC) study, 86 million adults aged 20 and over have pre-diabetes. That number is staggering, representing more than one in three US adults; unfortunately, it's even higher today!

Diabetes can be silent and sneaky, often undiscovered until other health issues get in our way.

Our HIGHLY processed food culture is designed to make us love food and crave things, hitting our bloodstream faster and raising our blood sugar. They are making us sicker than ever!

I say it's a blessing in disguise because... A pre-diabetes diagnosis allows you to alter your lifestyle course to a healthier, safer path.

On the other hand, if no changes are made... a complete diabetes diagnosis can mean blood sugar monitoring, taking drugs, and more doctor's appointments in your future, AT BEST.

The goal should be to make changes before you "have to;" it comes with less pressure on your terms and in your own time.

Romans 12:1 I beseech you therefore, brethren, by the mercies of God, that ye present your bodies a living sacrifice, holy, acceptable unto God, [which is] your reasonable service.

You can take control by:

- Eating less processed food. Adding more whole foods, fruits, vegetables, and whole grains.

- Eating fewer desserts.

- Cutting down on processed/refined sugar.

- If you're feeling hungry? Drink a glass of water, grab a piece of fruit or a palmful of nuts, and enjoy.

- Also, move more! Even a few minutes an hour could make a positive difference.

- AND... Don't be afraid to ask for help, ideas, or support from professionals or supportive friends and family members.

I want to share with you this universal challenge I saw on WebMD. What is just one thing you could add or one choice you could make a little differently that would support your health this week? Whatever that is, Give it a try and see how you feel. They added: "Perhaps one change isn't going to change everything. But one change at a time can!"

So, let's begin and prepare for a "You are not pre-diabetic" diagnosis at your next doctor's visit!

I pray that this message has been a blessing to you. Share this information with friends and family and share the good news that living fit offers.

Be blessed!

Arthritis

Arthritis. What is it? And how can we avoid or manage it?

The Centers for Disease Control (CDC) Reported 2013 and 2015, Approximately (22.7%) of 54.4 Million US Adults were told they have some form of arthritis:

Rheumatoid, Gout, Lupus, or Fibromyalgia

And... that figure is projected to be 63 Million by 2020 and 67 million by 2025.

So, what is arthritis?

Well, our bodies are designed to protect themselves. Inflammation in our bodies is a normal function that protects us from infection and foreign substances, such as bacteria and viruses.

However, arthritis occurs when the body triggers inflammation when there are no foreign substances in our body to fight off... we call this an autoimmune disease, which damages the body, causing pain, swelling, and stiffness.

Arthritis, primarily, comes from the foods we eat!

So, if we can control the type of food we eat, we can control whether or not we get arthritis.

On the other hand, if we continue to eat poorly, we will continue to suffer.

Yes, there are many drugs on the market that will make you look and feel better, but there is no medical cure for arthritis, and the drugs... doctors prescribe have side effects, and some of them cause death.

So, although you may look and feel better, initially, ultimately, the problem is still there.

You can reduce the symptoms and even eliminate all traces of arthritis simply by eating or removing the right foods.

Three examples of anti-inflammatory foods are...

1. Whole Grains:

Oats and wheat offer fiber and essential vitamins and minerals. Fiber reduces inflammation.

2. Green, Leafy Vegetables, for example, spinach & kale, have anti-inflammatory properties.

3. Vitamin C found in oranges and other citrus fruits combat inflammation as well.

Three examples of inflammatory foods are...

1. ASPARTAME (Asper-TAME), a sugar substitute in many low-calorie drinks. People drink these drinks to lose weight. However, aspartame is known to trigger inflammation.

2. Gluten is known **to ignite inflammation.**

AND finally...

3. Saturated Fats, like those found in animal products such as bacon, steak, and milk, are NOTORIOUSLY known to induce inflammation.

"Why spend money on what is not bread, and your labor on what does not satisfy? Listen, listen to me, and eat what is good, and you will delight in the richest of fare."

- Isaiah 55:2.

Let's stop wasting our money on non-nutritious foods & doctors' bills and begin investing and healing ourselves by buying healthy foods AND relying less... on medications... that we know, have detrimental side effects.

I pray that this message has been a blessing to you. Share this information with friends and family.

Be blessed!

Unclog Arteries Naturally

"The eye is the lamp of the body. If your eyes are healthy, your whole body will be full of light.

But if your eyes are unhealthy, your whole body will be full of darkness. If then the light within you is darkness, how great is that darkness."

- Matthew 6: 22-23.

Clients are always asking, what can I do to ensure my blood work numbers come back good at my upcoming Dr. Appt.?

And, of course, my answer is always... you cannot OUTRUN or outwork a bad diet.

But, there are things you can do consistently to keep yourself healthy, that will contribute to good health, and thus good numbers.

RIGHT NOW... The biggest killer on our planet is, by far, heart disease, not COVID-19 or any other virus. Heart disease is responsible for a **quarter** of all deaths every year. This is according to statistics gathered by **The Centers for Disease Control and Prevention**.

Now, You might be wondering why heart disease is so deadly. Well, it's due to the buildup of plaque within your arteries.

This plaque buildup is more dangerous than the plaque buildup in your teeth because the space is smaller, and as plaque builds, it narrows the inner walls of your arteries, which leads to clogs that will stop the flow of blood.

Your arteries are blood vessels that send **oxygen-filled blood** from your heart to **all areas** of your body, including your skin and organs.

If you allow plaque to build up...you are hindering your blood flow, which can lead to an abundance of health issues.

So today, I'm going to give you **TWO GREAT foods that will naturally clear your arteries**. They are easy to add to any meal plan, **AND**... you can eat them every day:

1. Asparagus

Asparagus is one of the best ways to cleanse your arteries. Eating asparagus will stimulate the production of healthy antioxidants; it is rich in various minerals and also holds high amounts of fiber. It can **prevent blood clots** and **lower your blood pressure**. **This will prevent most cardiovascular issues.** It can also relieve any **inflammation** in your body which might otherwise cause heart issues if left untreated.

Asparagus also contains **folic acid,** which will **prevent any hardening within your arteries**. And it is rather tasty!

2. Eat Avocado

Avocado is another green food that can help your arteries stay healthy. There are two types of cholesterol. There's good cholesterol (HDL) and bad cholesterol (LDL). When you eat avocado, it lowers the levels of bad cholesterol in your body and increases the levels of good cholesterol, thus clearing out your arteries. It also has high levels of vitamin E, which will prevent cholesterol oxidation.

Also, it has been known for centuries that avocados contain potassium, which has been an effective way to lower blood pressure.

Avocados are also very tasty food and can be eaten as a substitute for mayonnaise, on your salads and sandwiches, and as a form of guacamole.

Both asparagus and avocados are **recommended by the American Heart Association (AHA).**

So there you have it... Let's keep those arteries unclogged and bring home good doctor reports to our families and ensure them that we will be around healthy for years to come...

I pray it has been a blessing. Share it with your family and friends, and remember to tune in to Living Fit with James and

Karen Roberts every Tuesday at 11 am on WLJF, 100.7 FM
The Joy!

Avoiding Inflammatory Illnesses

Inflammatory illnesses include arthritis, osteoporosis, and most joint pains.

If you are having problems walking, reaching, bending, or any other kind of joint problem, then this message is for you.

If you tell your doctor that you are having trouble walking, climbing stairs, tying your shoes, or, you have some hard knots in some of your joints, for example, by your wrists. The doctor may tell you that you have BONE SPURS... deterioration, calcium deposits, arthritis, osteoporosis, or that it's part of the natural aging process or even hereditary.

Basically, the doctor is telling you that you have inflammation in your body!

If you ask how this happened... if they're not educated in nutrition, they may not know the answer, or they'll give you a calcium prescription, potion, lotion, pill, or recommend surgery as a temporary fix.

However, our bones and joints are made to last a lifetime without those fixes.

Inflammation PRIMARILY comes from the foods we eat.

There are specific foods that have an acid effect on the body, thereby causing a leak of minerals out of our bones, i.e. they deplete the body of calcium and other minerals.

Studies show that many people living in RN homes, who have osteoporosis, are often treated with calcium supplements, yet they still have osteoporosis; why is this?

Well, for one thing, if they eat meat (red/white), dairy, hybridized wheat, drink caffeine, and/or use tobacco, they are supplying their blood with acid-forming foods.

So, the lungs/kidneys begin to work overtime to restore proper acidic balance to the body, and in the process, begin to wear out.

Calcium is then released to neutralize the acid, restoring the blood levels back to normal…

But this comes at a COST; the calcium comes from the bones…

The excess calcium in the blood appears AS "Bone SPURS"…

I'M SURE YOU'VE HEARD OF… GOUT, ARTHRITIS, KIDNEY STONES, AND GALlSTONES… that's where they come from.

"Do not be wise in your own eyes;
fear the Lord and shun evil."
"This will bring health to your body
and nourishment to your bones."

- *Proverbs ch. 3 7-8.*

Most People think calcium builds bones, but that is just a small percentage of the reality. Bones are built with 12 minerals (One of them being calcium), and 64 trace minerals. Calcium gets the crown because the other minerals piggyback upon the calcium as it is distributed throughout the body. Without the other 11 minerals and trace minerals, we have the epidemic of osteoporosis that we have now.

The good news is, that we can prevent these inflammatory illnesses by eating the highest minerals nature has to offer, such as sunflower seeds and tahini butter, which are number one for supplying the body with calcium, followed by organic foods and veggies, including dark leafy greens.

So do yourself a favor; if you want to avoid inflammatory illnesses, I suggest,

- Workout with resistance training
- Eat clean and healthy foods

- Drink plenty of water

And if possible, make sure you are sleeping between 9 pm – 2 am. That's the primary time when the body **regenerates itself**.

Thank you, and remember to pass this on to friends and family.

Be blessed!

Getting Rid Of High Cholesterol

The Bible says:

"And he said to his disciples, "Therefore I tell you, do not be anxious about your life, what you will eat, nor about your body, what you will put on."

(ESV) Luke 12:22.

Between 2015-16, the CDC found that 50% of men aged 60 years and older were taking medication to lower cholesterol. Among women, the figure was 38%. Today, that number is even higher.

And current studies show Americans are being diagnosed at a younger and younger age.

Cholesterol is a waxy substance that is found in the fats in your blood. While your body needs and can make cholesterol to continue building healthy cells, having high cholesterol can increase your risk of heart disease.

When you have high cholesterol, you may develop fatty deposits in your blood vessels. Eventually, these deposits make it difficult for enough blood to flow through your arteries. This could lead to a heart attack or stroke.

There are NO symptoms of high cholesterol. A blood test is the only way to determine if you have high cholesterol.

Some of the risk factors that you should be aware of include:

- Poor diet
- Obesity
- Having a large waist circumference
- Lack of exercise
- Smoking
- And being diabetic

These risk factors could lead to

- Chest pain
- Heart attack
- Or stroke

So, what steps can we take to reduce high cholesterol?

1. Eat a low-salt diet that includes many fruits, vegetables, and whole grains.
2. Limit the number of animal fat you consume. Choose good fats like nuts and avocados.

3. Exercise on most days of the week for at least 30 minutes. Set a goal to reach a healthy weight for your height, and make sure your waistline is not wider than your hips. This is key to keeping diseases at bay!

4. Also, quit smoking and drinking, especially if you have a family history of HC.

God wants us to trust him. And as Christians, that means not being anxious for the things of this world. We all know God performs miracles, but how many of you know that miracles involve something that we can't do on our own?

If you notice, most "solutions" to current illnesses have the same remedy: eat healthily and work out. Now, is it easy? Some days, yes, others, no. The key is being consistent.

God wants us to do our part, because it shows obedience, and **that is** what GOD REALLY WANT'S FROM US!!!

I pray that this message has been a blessing to you. If you know anyone struggling with any of these conditions, please share this information with THEM!!! And as always, remember to tune into a living fit with James and Karen Roberts today at 11 am on WLJF 100.7 FM.

Be Blessed!

Four Ways To Eliminate Or Avoid High Blood Pressure

By making the following four lifestyle changes, you can lower your blood pressure and reduce your risk of heart disease.

Lifestyle plays a vital role in treating high blood pressure. Controlling blood pressure with a healthy lifestyle might prevent, delay, or reduce the need for medication.

Here are some lifestyle changes provided by the Mayo Clinic that can lower blood pressure and keep it down.

1. Lose Extra Pounds And Watch Your Waistline

Blood pressure often increases as weight increases. Being overweight also can cause disrupted breathing while you sleep (sleep apnea), which further raises blood pressure.

Weight loss is one of the most effective lifestyle changes for controlling blood pressure and many other diseases. If you're overweight or have obesity, losing even a small amount of weight can help reduce blood pressure. In general, blood pressure might go down by about one millimeter of mercury (mm Hg) with each kilogram (about 2.2 pounds) of weight lost.

Also, the size of the waistline is important. Carrying too much weight around the waist can increase the risk of high blood pressure.

In general:

• Men are at risk if their waist measurement is greater than 40 inches (102 centimeters).

• Women are at risk if their waist measurement is greater than 35 inches (89 centimeters).

2. Exercise Regularly

Regular physical activity can lower high blood pressure by about 5 to 8 mm Hg. It's important to keep exercising to keep blood pressure from rising again. As a general goal, aim for at least 30 minutes of moderate physical activity every day.

Exercise can also help keep elevated blood pressure from turning into high blood pressure (hypertension). For those who have hypertension, regular physical activity can bring blood pressure down to safer levels.

Some examples of aerobic exercise that can help lower blood pressure include walking, jogging, cycling, swimming, and dancing. Also, high-intensity interval training and strength training also can help reduce blood pressure.

3. Reduce Salt (Sodium) In Your Diet

Even a small reduction of sodium in the diet can improve heart health and reduce high blood pressure by about 5 to 6 mm Hg.

The effect of sodium intake on blood pressure varies among groups of people. In general, limit sodium to 2,300 milligrams (mg) a day or less. However, a lower sodium intake — 1,500 mg a day or less — is ideal for most adults.

To reduce sodium in the diet:

• **Read food labels.** Look for low-sodium versions of foods and beverages.

• **Eat fewer processed foods.** Only a small amount of sodium occurs naturally in foods. Most sodium is added during processing.

• **Don't add salt.** Use herbs or spices to add flavor to food.

• **Cook.** Cooking lets you control the amount of sodium in the food.

4. Get A Good Night's Sleep

Poor sleep quality — getting fewer than six hours of sleep every night for several weeks — can contribute to hypertension. A number of issues can disrupt sleep…Try to…

- **Stick to a sleep schedule.** Go to bed and wake up at the same time each day. Try to keep the same schedule on weeknights and on weekends.

- **Create a restful space.** That means keeping the sleeping space cool, quiet, and dark. Do something relaxing in the hour before bedtime. That might include taking a warm bath or doing relaxation exercises. Avoid bright light, such as from a TV or computer screen.

- **Watch what you eat and drink.** Don't go to bed hungry or stuffed. Avoid large meals close to bedtime. Limit or avoid nicotine, caffeine, and alcohol close to bedtime, as well…and finally,

- **Limit naps.** For those who find napping during the day helpful, limiting naps to 30 minutes earlier in the day might help nighttime sleep.

I pray this message has been a blessing to you; please pass it on to family and friends.

Some information in the section is complements of the Mayo Clinic

Be blessed.

Chapter 3 - Exercise

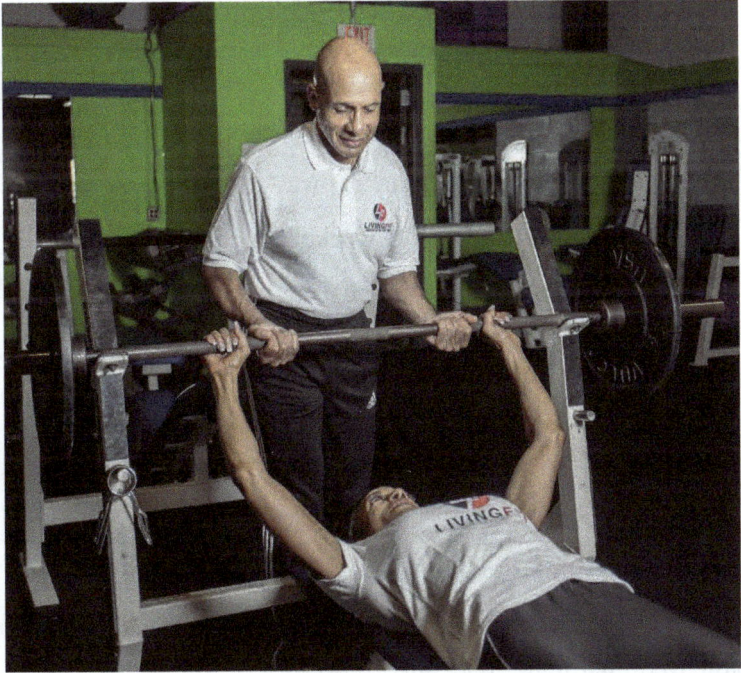

James (My husband) and I working out together. Working out with a partner has many benefits, including the ability to hold each other accountable.

Exercise Swaps To Build A Leaner Body

Working out has its pros. You can lose weight, get leaner, build endurance, and build an overall healthier body. Like many things, working out can have cons as well. For example, after doing the same exercises for weeks or even months on end, the body adapts to the workout, and progress can be stalled. The body needs to be challenged in order to change, and that requires constantly changing your workout about every four to eight weeks, depending on your goals. A simple swap of one exercise for another similar exercise can make all the difference in your fitness program.

Swap #1: Squats For Step-Ups

Squats are a functional movement that the body should be able to do naturally. We squat to do a lot of things, like tie our shoes, pick up bags and laundry, and more. Squats are a multi-functional movement, working the lower back, glutes, quadriceps, hamstrings, hips, knees, and ankles, and even contribute to flexibility. Squats can be performed just about everywhere, and you don't even need any equipment.

Step-ups use basically the same muscles, plus they add an element of cardio.

How to perform a step-up:

You will need a sturdy bench, stool, or box. Stand hip-width apart, with toes pointing forward, lift one foot, and put it on the box. Make sure your whole foot is on the box, not just your toes. Be sure to keep your foot, knee, and hip in alignment. Use the leg on the box (the front leg) to drive your body up while keeping your posture upright. Then, step down using the back leg. Try to avoid rocking as it could put undue pressure on your knees and unwillingly take the glutes and abdominals out of the exercise.

As you get stronger, you can add some dumbbells or a weight bar, and you can make the box/bench higher for an added level of endurance.

Swap #2: Push-Ups For Plank-Ups

Push-ups are one of the hardest yet most effective exercises to get the body in shape. They work your entire upper body, including your core, and they even work your glutes and quadriceps.

Swap out plank-ups for an incredible arm workout, and like push-ups, they work your entire body.

How to perform plank-ups

Start in a raised plank position, with your hands on the floor, directly under your shoulders. Keep your body in a straight line. Do not allow your hips to dip towards the floor, or raise to the ceiling. Keep your abdominals and glue muscles tight. Bend one elbow, bringing it to the floor/mat, then repeat with the other arm. Then, raise back up to the starting position one arm at a time. That would be one rep.

Perform four sets of 10-12 reps twice a week for great results.

Swap #3: Standard Lunges for Curtsey Lunges

The lunge is a multi-joint exercise, like the squat, that strengthens the entire lower body. Lunges also help to strengthen your core and improve hip flexibility, which can strengthen the lower back.

The curtsey lunge works the entire lower body. It also stabilizes the hips and works and tones the glutes.

How to Perform a curtsey lunge:

Start with a shoulder-width stance. Take the right foot and circle it around and behind the left foot. Going slightly past the left leg. At this point, you may clasp your hands together or keep them out by your sides for balance. Next, lunge down as deeply as possible, reaching the knee towards the floor. Slowly return to the starting position. Then, take the left foot and repeat the movement.

Perform three sets of 10 curtsey lunges. Doing each leg one time is one rep. Perform three sets of 10 curtsey lunges.

Walking Backward

I have a little Challenge for you; It's called "Walking BACKWARD."

Bible Verse:

"Therefore, strengthen your feeble arms and weak knees. "Make level paths for your feet," so that the lame may not be disabled, but rather healed."

- Hebrews 12:12-13.

Discipline is a tool used to help us grow and mature into the people God designed us to be. It is a method of correcting, strengthening, guiding, and healing us so that we are able to follow the righteous path the Lord has given us.

Exercising does the same thing.

Each day we unconsciously put one foot in front of the other, going about our way, not giving what we're doing a second thought. Since we are so used to walking forward, it may be tough to suddenly start trying to walk backward.

So, why should we walk backward?

Well, here are some of the health benefits of walking backward:

It:

- Improves coordination

- adds variety to your training

- strengthens leg and glute muscles

- decreases lower back pain

- puts less strain on the knees

- speeds up the metabolism

- increases energy level

- improves sleep

- strengthens the heart… and

- challenges the body with a different exercise.

Which In turn,

- strengthens the brain muscle.

As mentioned before, as you get comfortable doing this exercise, you can add weight (dumbbells or a bar) and begin to jog or skip to make it more challenging. If you are uncomfortable walking backward on the street, practice first on a treadmill or a wide-open area until you feel confident enough to go on your own.

Stay focused, watch your balance, and make sure the coast is clear. Be sure there are no people or objects behind you.

This is an awesome way to strengthen both your body and your brain at the same time!

Please share this information with your family and friends.

And be blessed!

Making Exercise A Daily Priority

"For where your treasure is, there will your heart be also."

- Luke 12:34.

If we say our bodies are the temple of God, we should be treating them in that manner.

So here are seven tips I hope will help you achieve that:

1. Make an appointment to exercise;

Put it on your calendar, and set your alarm for each day to do something (at home or the gym) until it becomes a habit.

2. Exercise in the morning;

There's no better feeling than starting your day having already done something successfully. And working out, no matter how long/short, is always a WIN! And it can set the tone for the rest of the day!

3. Cater to your likes and dislikes;

If you don't like doing the elliptical, taking group classes, or rowing machines, don't do it! Find something you want to do that you like. Go for a walk or ride a bike. Because if you like it, chances are you'll do it!

4. Make it social;

Recruit family members or friends to join in.

5. Boost activity throughout the day;

You can do many things throughout the day to increase your activity level and boost your step count, such as taking the stairs or parking farther from your destination and then walking. All of these activities add up as calories burned.

6. Workout efficiently;

Plan your workout ahead of time so you are not aimlessly walking around and wasting time. One of the most common excuses is that they have no time to work out! You will find that having a plan and sticking to it will get you in and out in no time. And you can go on with the rest of your day or evening.

7. And my favorite, set a goal, track your progress, and reward yourself;

For e.g. I keep a log of my workouts. I try to do just a little more than I did the previous week. Whether it's getting there 10 min earlier, lifting a few pounds heavier, or doing an extra set. And over time, If I was successful, I may reward myself with something healthy and usually not food-related. It could be something simple, like a new workout t-shirt.

The main idea here is to make exercising a priority and part of your daily routine or lifestyle. It is the same as honoring God by praying and studying the word!

Remember, our bodies are the temple of God; let's treat them that way!

I pray that this message has been a blessing to you. Share this information with friends and family.

Be blessed!

Spiritual Benefits From Exercising

Romans 12:1 says, Therefore, I urge you, brothers and sisters, in VIEW of God's mercy, to offer *your* bodies as a Living Sacrifice holy and pleasing to God... this is your true and proper worship.

God has many expectations of us, and exercising is one of them. We must exercise our bodies, mind, and spirit to remain functional in all areas!

Exercise does not benefit us just from the neck down; Exercise gives us a fresh supply of blood and oxygen to the brain. This clears the mind of stress, anxiety, depression, sadness, and anger.

With everything going on all around us, from COVID to climate change to environmental challenges and wars, exercising is exactly what we need to be doing.

Reading the Bible, meditating, and focusing on prayer will give the body a mental and spiritual lift. A well-functioning brain offers many benefits, from being sensitive to the needs of those around us to being sensitive to God's voice!

Have you ever read a bible verse and realized you didn't understand what you read? Or have you ever called yourself doing a good deed and later realized that God told you to do something else? An example would be buying someone groceries when God told you to give them the money.

By exercising our brains, we can optimize how we function spiritually.

Another aspect of this is that we need to take care of our physical beings.

And I'm not referring to how cute or strong we are!

"And the Lord God took the man and put him into the Garden of Eden to dress it and to keep it."

- Genesis 2:15.

In other words, we had to WORK.

As Christians, we should be prepared for anything God calls us to do.

We are meant to be active!

A strong body gives us the ability to help others in ways they can't help themselves.

It also aids our body in removing toxins and waste that clog our organs and make us TOO slow to react, TOO sick to help others, and TOO tired to move.

If we resort to lying around and remaining inactive, our muscles and organs atrophy... become WEAK... thereby allowing the illness to invade our bodies Like weeds invade an unattended GARDEN!... Or how COVID/flu attacks a weak body.

In Exodus 20:8, God commands his people to work six days and rest on the 7th.

"And this happened way back in the Garden of Eden even before Adam and Eve sinned."

- Genesis 2:3.

In general, we all need to eat and drink healthy and, as much as possible, get outside and be active. Become a volunteer, or:

- Mow your yard, or better yet, help mow someone else's yard!

- Help someone paint their fence or house

- Do some community service,

There are hundreds, if not thousands, of ways to be active.

I often tell my clients that you don't have to go to the gym to get exercise. But you do need to move your body.

These things will give you more brain clarity, a functioning body, and a sense of purpose, and they will show you as holy and pleasing to God!

I pray that this message has been a blessing to you. Share this information with friends and family.

How To Obtain A Flat Stomach

Our bodies are to be stirred up, exercised, and improved, lest they should be lost or taken away...

"For physical training is of some value, but godliness has value for all things, holding promise for both the present life and the life to come."

— 1 Timothy 4:8.

When I ask my clients which body part they want to get lean the most, it is almost always the stomach.

If you feel your stomach area is a problem, you are not alone. This is typical of people who have given birth or have already lost weight but want to get leaner.

So here's what I can tell you...

Focusing solely on your stomach is the same as target training, and as I said previously, you can't pick the actual area in which you want to lose fat. No one has a flat stomach, 24/7. Everyone's waistline (and body in general) fluctuates from time to time, even the leanest people. But you can get a slimmer, leaner stomach by following some of the tips below:

1. Add some total body workouts 2-3 times a week. And make sure you keep the intensity as high as "YOU" can handle. It's almost like high-intensity interval training (HIIT). This will result in more calories burned, overall body fat loss, and less time spent in the gym.

2. Get your core strong - One of the best exercises you can do to strengthen your core is a plank.

Not only do planks improve your core, but they help improve balance and strengthen your back, chest, and even legs. And when strengthening the core, don't forget to work your obliques. This will help your overall toning and give you a great-looking waistline.

And,

3. Stay away from alcohol and added sugar, and take control of your eating habits - not only is alcohol full of empty calories, but it releases estrogen into the bloodstream, which in excess can cause you to put on weight which can manifest outside the body, and on the inside (as fatty liver disease).

There's a saying: You can't outrun a bad diet. You want to get rid of all processed foods, microwave dinners and snacks (e.g. Popcorn), fast foods, chips, and soda...because they pile on the extra sugar and sodium and will indeed prevent you from getting a flat stomach.

Try eating whole foods, fruits, vegetables, lean proteins, and heart-healthy fats. Drink plenty of water… it will prevent bloating, boost your metabolism, and contribute to your overall better health and wellness!

"Guard, through the Holy Spirit who dwells in us (meaning our bodies)*, the treasure which has been entrusted to you."*

— 2nd Timothy 1:14.

Obtaining a flat stomach and optimum health depends on practicing good lifestyle habits; you can do this.

I pray that this message has been a blessing to you. Share this information with friends and family.

Be blessed!

How To Build Firm Glutes

5 Tips To Firm Up Your Glutes

If you're not happy with the way your glutes look and want to tighten and tone them, then read on!

The way to firm up your glutes starts with eating healthy and being consistent in your glute workouts. The glutes are made up of three muscles: the gluteus maximus, gluteus medius, and gluteus minimus. Here are some glute tips to help you sculpt a round, lean gluteus maximus:

Barbell Hip Thrust

The barbell hip thrusts activate the lower back, upper thigh, and butt. To perform this exercise, you need a bench or chair. Sit on the floor with your back against the chair/bench and your legs extended in front of you. Place the barbell across your lap. Rest your shoulders on the bench, squared and aligned to the bar. Lean back, keep those shoulders straight, and squeeze your glutes as you bring your hips upwards to the ceiling, lifting the bar. Really engage those glutes by squeezing them together as you do this lift. Take a moment at the top to hold the barbell up before you slowly hinge your hips to return to the starting position. Keep your neck straight throughout the movement.

Perform three sets of 15 reps twice a week.

The Romanian Deadlift

You will need a barbell or pair of dumbbells (a weight you can handle without losing your form). Start with the weight at your feet, and lift it to hip level- keeping your arms locked, your shoulders tucked back, and your neck/spine straight. Raise up to a straight position with your arms locked down. Slowly bend to lower the bar down to your lower calf as you continue to hold your spine straight. Pull your hips forward to bring the bar back up, and repeat for three sets of 15 reps.

Fire Hydrants

This exercise requires you to start on all fours. If this is too difficult to do on the floor, you may use a bench or mat, kneeling on all fours. Place shoulders so they are directly above your hands, with your hips directly above your knees. Keep your neck out straight, looking directly at the floor. Lift one leg out to the side, leading with your knee. Bring it up to a 45-degree angle. Slowly bring that back to your body. Do 15 reps on one leg, then the other.

Do three sets of 15 reps twice a week.

Dumbbell Walking Lunges

Walking lunges is like doing a whole-body workout. Hold a dumbbell in each hand, shoulders back, and arms straight; step forward with one leg, dropping the back knee towards the floor until you are at a 90-degree angle or parallel to the floor.

Pause for a few seconds at the bottom before lifting up to move the back leg forward and drawing to the same angle with the opposite knee. Keep moving forward for 10-20 alternating reps. A step forward on each leg is one rep. Repeat for three to four sets twice a week.

Donkey Kickbacks

Once again, start this exercise by getting on all fours; the elbows should be under your shoulders, clasp the fingers in front of you on the mat, the knees should be under your hips, keep your core tight, and you may tuck your toes. Lift one leg, pressing the heel of that foot toward the ceiling. Do not shift weight to one side or arch your back. Then, return back down to the mat (starting position).

After doing 15 on one leg, do the same on the other, and that would be one set. Add leg weights to make it more challenging.

Be Blessed!

How To Build Strong, Lean, And Toned Shoulders

The fact that Jesus came to Earth in a human body and not as an animal further demonstrates God's regard for our physical beings. In the Bible, Paul tells believers bluntly that their bodies are from God; therefore, believers should honor God with their bodies (1 Corinthians 6:20).

I feel we are called to steward our bodies as temples of the Holy Spirit. Therefore, if we do not show care for our health, we are neglecting God's temple.

As a certified trainer, I know combining cardio, strength training, and a healthy diet is a great way to reduce body fat.

When it comes to sculpting strong, defined shoulders, I feel one of the most effective exercises is the lateral raise. Not only will they give you great-looking shoulders, but as one of the most used joints in the body, the lateral raise will strengthen the joints, reducing the chance of injury.

To perform a lateral raise, you may stand or sit. Hold a weight in each hand, and keep feet shoulder-width apart for stability. The arm should be at your side, at a 90-degree angle, with palms facing in. Keep the elbow in line with the shoulder and wrist in line with the elbow (a 90-degree angle). Slowly raise your arms out to the side, Keeping the same alignment throughout the entire movement. Stopping at shoulder height. Then, slowly bring the arms back to the starting position. That is one rep. Do three to four sets of 10-15 reps once to twice a week for awesome-looking shoulders.

Pass this information to friends and family, and be blessed.

Awesome Tricep Exercises

Bible Verse:

"Your eye is the lamp of your body. When your eye is healthy, your whole body is full of light. But when it's evil, your body is full of darkness."

- Luke 11:34.

As we get older, gain weight, or both, we begin to notice things about our bodies, whether or not we work out. One of the things we notice is extra skin hanging off the back of our arms. If you are in this category, you are not alone. But no worries, most people can tone and build muscle on the back of their arms just by adding a few easy tricep exercises and doing them consistently, once or twice a week.

The triceps (opposite the bicep) are a group of three muscles on the back of your arm that go from your shoulder to your elbow. They're used for fine motor skills like playing tennis, doing push-ups, and throwing a baseball to doing household chores, like sweeping the floor and vacuuming.

Remember, solely targeting the tricep will not give you skinny, sculpted arms (if that is your goal). But building your tricep muscles as an overall part of your workout routine does benefit you in that it adds toneness, makes other upper body exercises easier, helps your body lose weight, and… muscle mass burns calories much faster than fat, and even it does so at rest.

Here are three ways to tone and shape the back of the arms with just a pair of dumbbells or even water bottles.

Tricep Extensions

The tricep extension is one of the simplest exercises you can do. However, it does require a little arm flexibility.

You can stand or sit:

- (Stands with your) Feet shoulder-width apart.

- Grab the weight with both hands. Lift the weight up and over your head. Then, lower the weight behind your head, holding it between your shoulder blades.

- Lift your arms so they're straight above your head and back down, making sure your elbows don't flare out and repeat.

- Aim for four sets of 12-15 reps one to two times a week.

Tricep Kickbacks

You will definitely feel this exercise on the back of your arm.

To Start:

- Stand with your feet together, knees slightly bent, and bent forward at the waist approximately at a 90-degree angle.

- Hold your weights with your arms hanging straight down, then pull the elbows back, pulling your hands towards your waist while keeping your arms close to your side. Your elbows and the back of your arms should be slightly higher than your back. That is your starting position.

- Then, press your forearms back until your arms are straight (hence the name kickback, because you're literally kicking your arms back) while keeping your elbows in the high starting position. Then, bring your forearms forward and repeat the press back. Repeat all reps before standing back up. Then, repeat for four sets for 12-15 reps.

Stay consistent, and you should see your arms tightening up in no time.

Tricep Dips

Dips are more of a challenge to the triceps because you're supporting your whole body. But they work amazingly well.

- You'll need a chair, table, or bench to sit on. Place your hands on it, shoulder-width apart, on either side of your hips.

- Put your feet in front of you with a slight bend in the knees.

- Scoot your glutes off the bench, keeping your back close to the bench. And then slowly bend your elbows, lowering your body toward the floor, until your elbow is at about a 90-degree angle.

- Once you reach the 'bottom' of the move, begin to push your weight back up until you're able to scoot your glutes back on the bench.

- To make it easier, bend your knees more and straighten your legs to make it more challenging.

- Do about three to four sets of 12-15 reps twice a week.

As always, I hope this has been a blessing to you. Remember to share this information with your friends and family.

Be blessed.

Biceps Exercises

The bicep brachii, better known as the bicep, is one of two muscles in the arm. The other is the tricep, which we just talked about. There are two parts to the bicep: the short head, and the long head. The main movement of the biceps is flexion at the elbow joint and supination (allowing you to curl upward) of the forearm.

The short head and long head of the biceps contract to help the arm flex or bend, for example, reaching out to give someone a hug.

There are many different bicep exercises you can incorporate into your workout regimen. Here are some I feel work the best.

Alternating Dumbbell Curls:

Stand with your feet shoulder-width apart. Keep your shoulders back and core tight. Grab the dumbbells with palms facing outward and slightly in front of your hips. Slowly curl one hand upward to ward the bicep, then lower it back to the starting position, then do the same with the other arm. Keep alternating until you have done ten reps for each arm, which will be one set.

Perform three to four sets of ten reps twice a week.

Incline Curls:

You will need an incline (Raise to about 45 - 60 degrees) bench or high-back chair. Grab your dumbbells and sit on the bench, leaning back with arms fully extended and palms facing outward. Elbows should be locked and behind your body to start. Keep your stomach tight, chest lifted, and feet flat on the ground in a comfortable position (wide or close). Slowly, simultaneously raise both hands up toward the bicep, then as you lower your arm back down, think of resisting the weight all the way down to the starting position. This would be one rep.

Perform three to four sets of ten reps once or twice a week.

Seated Concentration Curls:

You will need a bench or chair for this exercise and just one dumbbell. Sit with feet wider than shoulder-width apart. Pick up the dumbbell with the left hand and lean over to place the left tricep (or back of your arm) onto the inside of the left thigh. Adjust your feet for width. Start with a full extension, just shy of locking out the elbow. Slowly begin to curl the weight up towards the shoulder, squeeze the biceps at the top and hold for a second, then lower the hand back to the starting position. Repeat ten times, then do the other arm for one complete set. Be sure not to rock back and forth or move your arm up and down while doing the exercise.

Perform three to four sets of 10-12 reps once or twice a week.

Be Blessed!

Why We Need And How To Maintain Healthy Feet

"Watch the path of your feet, and all your ways will be established."

- Proverbs 4:26

There are only 26 small bones in your feet, and they carry the weight of your entire body.

Feet are vital to walking, skipping, jumping, running, and more. However, you may not think to train and strengthen your feet like you'd approach other body parts. Ignoring your foot muscles can lead to weakness and lack of flexibility, which may result in injuries and even pain.

As we age, our body naturally begins to lose flexibility. If we stand idle and do nothing, we could be less able to absorb the stress our daily activities require. For example, doing daily exercises, walking up and down the stairs, and even just walking up and down the aisles of a store could be difficult or even painful without flexible feet and ankles. If your foot and ankle cannot sufficiently absorb that shock, you'll likely experience increased strain throughout your knee and hip. Weak feet may create ankle, knee, and hip problems down the road.

Also, foot issues could cause you to compensate for the problem in some way, which usually means a loss of mobility or strength in those other areas. This can cause you to develop a limp or can lead to joint problems and low-back issues as well."

One of the best things we can do for our bodies is to maintain flexibility, especially as we age.

In searching for a great exercise to strengthen the feet, I came across an exercise called the towel roll. This exercise not only strengthens the foot but also increases flexibility, improves the range of motion, and improves everything from the toes all the way up the leg to the hamstrings and glutes.

Here's how to perform it:

-Sit in a chair on a hard surface floor (not a rug).

-Place a small hand or dish towel on the floor.

-Put your foot on the towel with your toes towards the front of the towel.

-Use your toes to grab the towel and pull it towards your heels without lifting your heels.

-Flare your toes and grab again, continuing to roll the towel until it is rolled up under your feet. Then, use your toes to unroll the towel. And do the same with the other foot.

Do three to four sets of five reps at least once a week or as often as needed to maintain foot strength and flexibility.

I pray that this message has been a blessing to you. Share this information with friends and family.

Be blessed!

Chapter 4 - Life Events

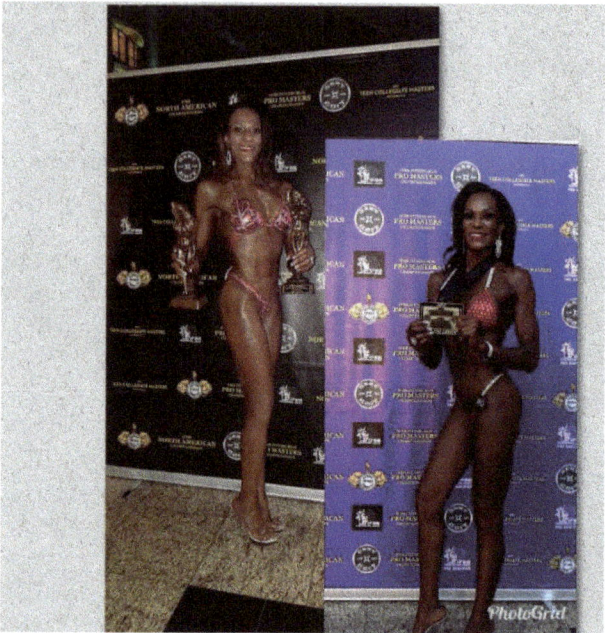

This is me after months of hard training and dieting and winning 2nd and 3rd place at an NPC National Bodybuilding Competition.

"Six" Components Of Living A Healthy Lifestyle

Living a healthy lifestyle is a saying that seems to be thrown around a lot. Well, What exactly does that mean? And why is it important?

Are your daily lifestyle choices setting you up for illness later in life, or even worse, are they making you sick right now?

Most people would say a healthy person generally:

- Does not smoke

- Maintains a healthy body weight

- Eats a balanced diet

- Practices self-love

- Has a positive attitude

- Exercises regularly, and

- Has good social circles (friends/family)

Also, many people associate wealth with health. And for good reason, because wealthy people, in many cases, have access to more/or better (perceived) options in general (Including medical care, healthy whole foods, etc.) versus people who are not as wealthy.

However, not only can money not buy life, but I've never seen any definitions of a healthy lifestyle that included the word money. Living healthy is not just the absence of disease, but it is the steps, strategies, and actions taken on purpose to achieve optimum health. In other words, you have to work for it!

Today, it is perceived as normal to live to a certain age and then spend the last 10 to 20 years suffering: Being sick, having operations, having multiple doctor's appointments, being put in rehab and nursing homes, and taking medications in many cases for life!

The reality is that we should be living right up until we die, meaning we should be enjoying all of the components of living healthy right up until we pass.

So, here are "six" "MUST HAVE" components that should help you live a healthy lifestyle.:

1. Trust in GOD because He gave us self-healing bodies. (a minor cut that healed itself)

2. Eat a healthy diet and be physically active (Refined sugar/feelings of sluggishness vs. unrefined carbs/feelings of energy).

3. Get adequate rest and manage stress (to maximize mental well-being).

4. Learn to forgive, love, and show compassion (to people/animals)

5. Laugh and be genuinely happy (especially with ourselves/self-love).

6. Having meaningful relationships with family and friends (a good social circle).

So why Is living a healthy lifestyle so important?

Because studies show, lifestyle plays a huge role in how healthy we are.

Currently, too many people are relying on doctors, pills, procedures, and technology to cure them of diseases acquired from living unhealthy lifestyles. Many diseases can be prevented or delayed just with simple lifestyle changes.

The Bible says:

"If you listen carefully to the LORD your God and do what is right in his eyes if you pay attention to his commands and keep all his decrees, I will not bring on you any of the diseases I brought on the Egyptians, for I am the LORD, who heals you."

– Exodus 15:26

Living a healthy lifestyle is simple but not easy! A great way to start is by using the list of 6 components I gave you as a check-off list and begin the journey to living a life dedicated to optimizing your health.

Be blessed!

Staying Injury Free During The Winter Season

Shoveling snow is rarely an easy task! It can be just as strenuous as a workout. You can burn 500 or more calories. And if you're not careful, you could end up with a severe injury to the back, severe muscle strain, frostbite, or a heart attack.

So here are eight tips to help you shovel injury-free:

1. You may want to consider getting some help or wearing a back brace

2. take frequent breaks and drink a warm beverage, especially if you're feeling cold or numb.

3. It is easier to pull muscles when it is frigid outside. Just like working out, you may want to warm up before you go outside.

4. Dress warmly in light clothes that will soak up any sweat, such as thermals, to prevent frostbite.

5. Make sure your extremities are protected because they are the most vulnerable. These are your ears, nose, fingers, and toes.

6. Each year, about 120,000 accidents occur as a result of snow and ice removal. Try to wear waterproof boots that have good traction.

7. Snow can be heavy, so try to Invest in a lightweight shovel.

8. And finally, to minimize your chances of injury, try pushing the snow, not lifting it, whenever possible; this way, you don't put much strain on your back.

You Can't Work Off A Bad Diet!

As well as being a Certified Personal Trainer, I am also a Certified Sports Nutritionist. And... I get a lot of diet-related questions every day.

The most popular question is...Can I out workout a bad diet?

And the answer is absolutely not! The obvious proof of that is all the people who go to the gym or workout regularly, and their physical characteristics remain the same, or they gain weight (fat) or get sick.

Personally, I'd love to eat a whole pizza and then go for a run or to the gym for a quick workout to burn it off.

But our bodies just don't work that way!

Don't get me wrong, you will burn calories during a workout. And the more intense the workout, the more calories you're likely to burn.

The thing people need to be aware of is that our bodies are made to burn different calories differently:

For example, It could take four hrs. to burn off a 3000-calorie burger and fries meal, vs. just minutes to burn off a 500-calorie plant-based meal or salad.

In other words, you would be working out all day long, trying to burn off all the calories consumed in a bad diet. And you'd probably still be unhealthy because the food itself causes more than just weight gain, like high blood pressure and clogged arteries. And mentioning clogged arteries, there is no amount of exercise you could do that would unclog your arteries. You have to eat your way back to good health. In other words, eating certain foods, like broccoli, will help unclog your arteries, not exercising.

To look at it another way, even in the best-case scenario, even if you were able to burn off all the calories you ate. You could still be unhealthy due to the fat in your arteries, in or around your stomach, and major organs.

So, it does matter what we eat. And it is very relevant to maintaining good health and a healthy weight.

The best solution is to eat healthy, preferably a plant-based diet, or if you are a meat eater, choose small portions (2-4 oz max. per day) and lean/organic foods whenever possible.

Once again, thank you for your interest. Share this information with family and friends, and have a blessed day!

Fitness Resolutions!

Some of the most popular New Year's resolutions are: I will lose x amount of pounds, start going to the gym, or engage in some other health-related journey. And it's been that way for many years.

God wants us to be in good health, to be able to work, and to uplift the body of Christ!

"God gave talents, for the equipping of the saints, for the work of ministry, for the edifying of the body of Christ."

- Ephesians 4:12

As far back as I could research, getting healthier has been a top three New Year's resolution.

Making New Year's resolutions are easy. **Keeping it, however, is hard**!

Why is that? Mainly, it's because we don't plan ahead. If 90% of us plan ahead, 50% would at least attempt to follow through, and half of those people, about 25%, will make it through most of January. And of that amount, half, about 12%, will make it into February, and by March, the number will dwindle down to about 2 to 6%.

Don't get me wrong, getting in shape is a great New Year's resolution. But you must have a plan of action.

Here's what happens when you don't have a plan:

The day after New Year's, many people head to the gym with no plan and no outline of goals, and this is what happens:

- You walk in the door, the front desk is crowded, people are trying to get information, and you have to wait your turn.

- Stress and frustration levels begin to rise, but somehow, you make it through the process.

- Now, you're with a representative who gives you information, provides a walk-through of the facility, and perhaps signs you up.

- So, now you're on your own.

- If it is crowded, you could find yourself overwhelmed, frustrated, waiting for machines, and feelings of wanting to leave begin to creep in.

Planning may not take away all the anxieties, but it could lighten the burden.

Here's what you could do:

1.   Decide if you want to join a traditional or smaller gym, get a personal trainer, or both. This may mean looking at several facilities. You may not want to jump on the first offer you're given.

2.   Do your research! Budget for it! For example, in some cases, you don't have to pay a gym membership fee if you have a trainer. You just pay the trainer.

3.   Get your mind right. Mentally, be prepared for these things to happen. In other words, be prepared to be in line, hear a sales pitch, and be prepared to read & a contract. So, make sure you're not on a tight schedule. Plan to be there for a few hours. And have a list of questions with you to optimize your time. If you're out sooner, that would be great!

4. If possible, get a free trial pass. Some offer one to two weeks. Go the time you would normally work out. Sometimes, what we see online may not be the same in person. This way, you can try out the equipment and see if you like the environment. It could be the crowd is too old/young for you, or they play the music really loud. Or perhaps the equipment is worn and torn, or half the equipment is broken. All of these things could be red flags and things to take into consideration before signing a contract.

5. When you are ready to work out, know what you want to do. It is important to start with realistic goals. It takes time to get and stay in shape. So start where you are, at your fitness level, and build from there, and I wish you much success!

Be blessed!

Tips For Living A Healthier Summer

There is no perfect healthy time of the year. Just as during the winter months, we must take measures to keep our immune system optimum so that we don't get sick; we have to do the same in the summer. It may be for different reasons, such as surviving much warmer climates, versus the cold, but we are looking for the same end result, great health!

Some of the top experts suggest doing the following things will tremendously improve your overall health:

Give Your Diet a Berry Boost

If you do one thing this summer to improve your diet, have a cup of mixed fresh berries -- blackberries, blueberries, or strawberries -- every day. They'll help you load up on antioxidants, which may help prevent damage to tissues and reduce the risks of age-related illnesses. Blueberries and blackberries are especially antioxidant-rich.

A big bonus: Berries are also tops in fiber, which helps keep cholesterol low and may even help prevent some cancers.

Get Dirty -- and Stress Less

To improve your stress level, plant a small garden, cultivate a flower box, or if space is really limited, plant a few flower pots around the house, on the terrace, or anywhere -- indoors or out, that could have space for a flower pot.

Just putting your hands in soil is "grounding." Grounding, also known as earthing, is when humans make an electrical connection to the Earth's energies. The simplest form involves walking barefoot in the grass, dirt, or sand. And when life feels like you're moving so fast your feet are barely touching the turf, being mentally grounded can help relieve physical and mental stress.

Floss Daily

You know you need to; now it's time to start. Floss every single day. Do it at the beach, while reading, or when watching TV -- and the task will breeze by.

Flossing reduces oral bacteria, which improves overall body health, and if oral bacteria is low, your body has more resources to fight bacteria elsewhere. Floss daily, and you're doing better than at least 85% of people.

Take a Vacation!

Improve your heart health: take advantage of summer's slower schedule by using your vacation time to unwind. And, it doesn't have to be elaborate.

Vacations have multiple benefits: They can help lower your blood pressure, heart rate, and stress hormones such as cortisol, which contributes to a widening waist and an increased risk of heart disease.

And don't stress if you can't take a whole week off. The health benefits associated with taking time off work apply to any length of time taken off. So go, and enjoy yourself.

Sleep Well

Resist the urge to stay up later during long summer days. Instead, pay attention to good sleep hygiene by keeping the same bedtime and wake-up schedule and not eating or drinking (other than water) within three hours of bedtime.

It's also a good idea to avoid naps during the day unless you take them every day at the same time, for the same amount of time. Rather than focusing on digesting the food you eat, your body will be able to repair and rebuild itself.

And there you have it, some super simple ways to boost your health this summer. Try one or try them all. They're so easy you won't even know they're good for you.

Be blessed!

How To Optimize Your Time

The Number one excuse Most people have for not working out or doing other important things is that "they don't have the time". This is also one of the reasons why many people fall short of reaching their New Year's resolution goals.

The big picture here is you have to find a better work-life balance. For example, if you want to join a church or charity organization, have time to exercise, be more involved in your family, go out on the weekends, or attend your child's after-school activities, you must learn to optimize your time,

Here are some tips to help you optimize your time:

Figure Out Your Goals:

- write a list of goals,

- break them into smaller tasks,

- focus on how to fit them into your schedule, according to importance (prioritize)

- Then stick to it and hold yourself accountable for any missed appointments.

"Making the best use of time, because the days are evil. Therefore do not be foolish, but understand what the will of the Lord is."

- Ephesians 5:16-17.

Keep Track Of Your Time

It can help to take a week or so to note how long it really takes you to do things. For example, how long does it really take to do the laundry, make breakfast, clean the house, or even write a term paper? Most people overestimate simple tasks like taking a shower and underestimate the time needed for bigger tasks such as going shopping for your food for the week. If you know approximately how you spend your time, you may be able to manage it better.

"How long will you lie there, O sluggard? When will you arrive from your sleep? A little sleep, a little Slumber, a little folding of the hands to rest, and poverty will come upon you like a robber and want it like an armed man." - Proverbs 6:9-11.

Schedule Your Day

Once you know just how long things take and what's most important start to plan things out. Write it on the calendar. Create a to-do list. Put it on iCloud, so you have it wherever you go, and be flexible. Do you get more done in the late afternoon or early morning? Do you like to have your evenings free to relax? Are you more likely to do yard work if you have a chunk of time to do it all at one time or spread it out over the course of a week? Think about what works best for you, and don't be afraid to change things up.

"Walk in wisdom towards Outsiders, making the best use of time."

- Colossians 4:5.

Just Start!

If you feel a strong urge to put things off, find a way to push past it and take even a small step forward. You'll feel better once you make a little progress and may soon find yourself in a real Groove, and that's because your attitude often comes from your **behavior** - - **and your results** rather than the other way around.

I can't tell you how many times I started to just pick up a few items and ended up cleaning a whole room.

Once you get into the motion of doing the thing that you know you need to do, your mind and your attitude begin to change, and you begin to feel at peace with yourself, knowing you did something you should have been doing anyway, thus allowing you to rest easy when it's all said and done.

"Do your best to present yourself to God as one approved, a worker who has no need to be ashamed, rightly handling the word of Truth."

I pray that this message has been a blessing to you. Please pass it on to your family and friends, and have a blessed day!

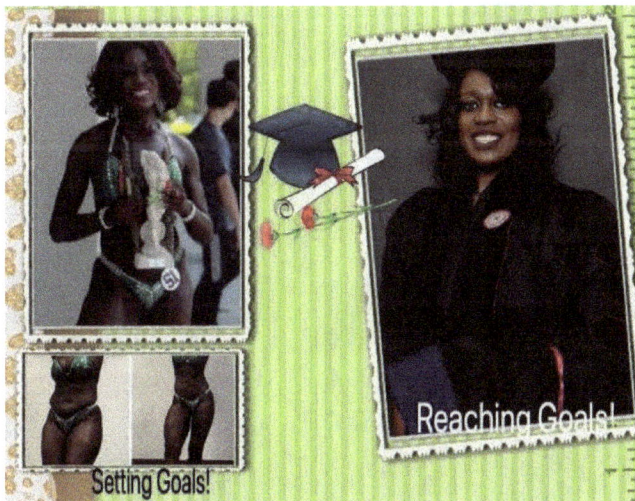

This is my client: Dr. Dianne Wellington. She never let daily life's struggles stop her from reaching her goals. From education to fitness, she always gives 100%.

Chapter 5 - Youth

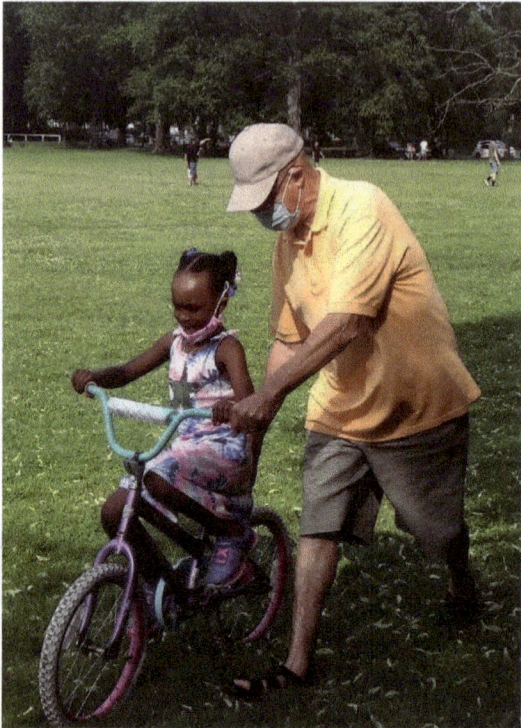

This is my Uncle Thomas, teaching my young cousin Serenity how to ride a bike: Being active as a child has immeasurable health benefits.

Childhood Diabetes Awareness

If you have type-1 diabetes, your pancreas doesn't make insulin or makes very little insulin. Insulin helps blood sugar enter the cells in your body for use as energy. Without insulin, blood sugar can't get into cells and builds up in the bloodstream. High blood sugar is damaging to the body and causes many of the symptoms and complications of diabetes.

Type-1 diabetes was once called insulin-dependent or juvenile diabetes. It usually develops in children, teens, and young adults, but it can happen at any age.

Type-1 diabetes is less common than type 2 — about 5-10% of people with diabetes have type-1.

Diabetes can be treated by following your health care specialists' recommendations for living a healthy lifestyle, which should include managing your blood sugar.

Type-2 diabetes is an autoimmune disease that mostly occurs in adults.

However, an article in USATODAY.COM states from 2000 to 2009, the prevalence of type-2 diabetes in children jumped more than 30%, to an astounding rate of 0.46 per 1,000 kids, according to a study presented at the Pediatric

Academic Societies meeting in Vancouver, Canada. And today, that number is even higher!

This disease causes the body to become resistant to the effects of insulin or doesn't make enough insulin, interfering with the absorption of blood glucose in the body.

Over time, having too much glucose in your blood can cause health problems, such as:

1. Heart disease and stroke

2. Kidney disease

3. Nerve damage

4. Amputation and

5. Vision loss… even in kids

If you suspect your child has diabetes, look for these six symptoms:

1. Excessive fatigue. If your child seems extremely tired or sleepy, changes in blood sugar may be affecting their energy levels.

2. Frequent urination

3. Excessive thirst

4. Increased hunger

5. Slow-healing sores

6. Darkened skin

Some of the main causes and risk factors are: overweight, obesity, and physical inactivity. Extra belly fat, in particular, is linked to insulin resistance and type-2 diabetes.

The symptoms often develop slowly—over months to several years—and can be so mild that you might not even notice them. Many people with type-2 diabetes have no symptoms. Some people do not find out they have the disease until they have a medical exam or diabetes-related health problems, such as blurred vision or heart trouble.

If you want to know if you have diabetes, there are two things you can do immediately:

1. Have the child's pediatrician check their Body Mass Index (BMI) at their next physical to determine if your child is at risk.

If it is too high, the doctor will let you know they are at risk, and what your options are.

2. Start building good gut bacteria in your child's body. You can do this by feeding your child a diet rich in vegetables and plant fiber.

Plant fiber encourages the growth of "GOOD" gut bacteria that help to break down and fight off diseases. Eating processed foods with little plant fiber reduces the good bacteria and increases the bad gut bacteria, making your child vulnerable to diseases.

> *"Train up a child in the way he should go; even when he is old he will not depart from it."*
>
> *- Proverbs 22:6.*

Remember, as Christians, we must lead by example and then teach these habits to our children.

Be blessed!

Childhood Obesity

In 1970, it was rare to see a child overweight. The obesity rate was around 6.1%. Today, that rate is over 20%; that's triple the number, and over 14 million children and adolescents are affected.

What are the leading causes of obesity?

The causes of obesity are varied and sometimes complex. However, studies show exposure to fast food ads, your environment, socioeconomic status, overeating and unhealthy snacking, and not getting enough exercise are all contributors. Americans are no strangers to obesity; around 90 percent of American adults fall into this category, according to the Centers for Disease Control and Prevention.

Here are some physical, social, and emotional risk factors you should be aware of:

a.   Poor diet – High-calorie foods, vending, sugary snacks, and sugary/fruity drinks.

b.   Lack of exercise – Too much sedentary time contributes greatly to obesity.

c.   Family-related – Coming from an overweight family. Contributing habits tend to be passed down from generation to generation.

d.   Psychological factors – Children tend to stress-eat, the same as adults.

e.   Socioeconomic factors – Accessibility to healthy foods and parks plays a key role.

The reason you need to be aware of these risk factors is that they can lead to physical complications such as

a. Type-2 diabetes – affects how the child's body uses glucose (sugar).

b.   Metabolic syndrome – causing heart disease, excess abdominal fat, or other health problems.

c.   High cholesterol and/or high blood pressure. A build-up of plaque in the arteries can lead to heart problems down the road.

d.   Asthma, sleep disorders, and non-alcoholic fatty liver.

e.   And finally, social and emotional problems, like Low self-esteem, being bullied, behavior/learning problems, and depression.

"So I have chosen him, that he may command his children and his household after him to keep the way of the Lord by doing righteousness and justice."

- Genesis 18:19

So, not only should we be eating clean and living a healthy lifestyle, but we are obligated to do so and to teach our children. As parents, grandparents, caretakers, and so on, we assumed the role of enablers. We buy the food and snacks and feed them to the children. Therefore, it is our responsibility to ensure our children have the healthiest foods possible.

Understanding that not everyone has access to the same food, however, the idea is to make better choices from what is available to you.

That being said, here's how we can fix it:

a. Limit your child's consumption of sugar-sweetened beverages.

b. Provide plenty of fruits and vegetables.

c. Eat meals as a family as often as possible.

d. Limit eating out (to birthdays and holidays), especially at fast food restaurants; Socialize at restaurants that serve healthy foods, not greasy spoons, and all-you-can-eat places, where the temptations are unlimited.

e. Adjust portion sizes appropriately for age.

f. Try to put yourself in healthy environments. Take hikes, go to the gym, and surround yourself with healthy-minded people.

g. And lastly, always follow up with your doctor, especially if you have health concerns.

Thank you, and have a terrific Tuesday.

Kids and Fatty Liver Disease

Years ago, alcoholic fatty liver disease was associated with adults due to heavy alcohol use. Your liver breaks down most of the alcohol you drink so it can be removed from your body, but the process of breaking it down can generate harmful substances. These substances can damage liver cells, promote inflammation, and weaken your body's natural defenses. The more alcohol that you drink, the more damage to your liver. Alcoholic fatty liver disease is the earliest stage of alcohol-related liver disease. The next stages are alcoholic hepatitis and cirrhosis.

Non-alcoholic fatty liver disease (NAFLD), a condition often associated with obesity, affects an estimated 80 million people in the United States and is the most common chronic liver condition in children and adolescents. It occurs when too much fat accumulates in the liver and triggers an inflammatory process that injures liver cells. It's generally symptomless, but as it progresses, fatty liver disease can interfere with critical liver functions.

With the rise in childhood obesity, more kids are developing the disease, and doctors are seeing more in their practices. Many parents are aware that obesity can lead to type-

2 diabetes and other serious metabolic conditions, but there is far less awareness of the link between obesity and liver disease.

NAFLD is diagnosed by measuring the blood levels of an enzyme called ALT, which is a marker for liver damage. But, it's difficult to diagnose the inflammatory component without a liver biopsy, so prevalence estimates are inaccurate. Autopsy studies suggest that about 1 in 10 children and adolescents have fatty liver, with or without inflammation, and that number is climbing.

In adults, the disease is a growing reason for liver transplants and, in some instances, liver cancer.

Cirrhosis—scarring of the liver due to chronic inflammation—is rare in kids, but it's a concerning long-term consequence that can lead to end-stage liver disease. Kids as young as six have been diagnosed with inflammation and even teens with cirrhosis.

The liver makes innumerable proteins, maintains the body's metabolism, and filters out toxins from our blood. The liver does not regenerate itself, like other parts of the body, so if it stops working, a liver transplant is the only treatment.

Studies show that three-year-olds with increased waist circumference had higher levels of ALT — a marker for liver damage — by the time they were eight. Those with greater increases in waist circumference and other measures of obesity also had higher ALT levels in their mid-childhood. This shows that we need to act early in a child's life to prevent excess weight gain and subsequent liver inflammation.

Besides losing weight, can anything else prevent or reverse non-alcoholic fatty liver disease?

Maintaining a healthy weight by eating more plant-based whole foods, fewer processed foods, and exercising regularly is the main way for kids and adults to prevent non-alcoholic fatty liver disease.

Studies suggest that eating recommended amounts of vitamin E — an antioxidant — may prevent liver inflammation. Foods that are rich in vitamin E include spinach, tomatoes, avocados, some types of fish, nuts, and seeds.

Vitamin E from supplements is absorbed differently than the dietary kind, so it's unclear if supplements could prevent liver inflammation. That's a study yet to be done.

Should children be screened for fatty liver disease?

Doctors have been indifferent about the screening efforts for NAFLD because there is no treatment other than weight loss, and there is no noninvasive screening tool. However, some clinicians measure ALT levels in all obese children starting at around age ten. This information can then be used to educate and guide parents to a healthy solution.

Health Habits For Kids

It's up to parents to teach their children the habits they need to live happy, healthy lives. Some of which can last a lifetime.

Consistency in what parents say and do is the key to teaching kids healthy habits. You can talk to a child all day long, but the reality is, kids mirror what they see. Especially from their parents, and that's why it is extremely important that parents practice what they preach. What's important to you will become important to them.

So here are five healthy habits parents can start teaching their kids right now:

1. Eat The Rainbow

Kids require a variety of nutrients to support growth and development. When choosing what to cook for your kids, make it a point to select fruits and vegetables with a variety of natural, bright colors. The richer/more vibrant the color, typically, the more nutritious, and stay away from juice and soda as much as possible.

2. Do Something Active Every Day

It's recommended that children get at least one hour of active play a day. If you're having trouble motivating your kids, try simple, affordable toys such as jump ropes, inflatable beach balls, and frisbees, and choose different locations to keep it fun and exciting—public parks and schools, playgrounds, baseball fields, and pools are all great options.

3. Take A Timeout From Devices

Research has shown that kids who cut down on TV watching and screen time also reduced their percentage of body fat, and it's pretty clear why. By limiting the time they spend in front of screens (including smartphones, tablets, and iPads), children have to find other activities to entertain themselves, such as participating in sports and other active games that promote creativity and physical exercise. And, as a bonus, less time in front of a screen means they can spend more time with you.

4. Keep Up With Check-Ups

In addition to ensuring all is well with your little one's health, these are opportunities for you to get invaluable advice on how to keep them well. These visits are also very important to make sure your infant or child is meeting their milestones appropriately. Be sure to keep a running list of questions so you don't forget to address these during your child's visit. In addition to regular visits with your primary care provider, be sure not to miss consistent dental and eye exams. Also, unless your doctor is the exception to the rule, most doctors get little, if any, nutritional education. So, if you have weight concerns, it may be helpful to ask your pediatrician to recommend a child nutritionist. This can be a game-changer.

The Benefits of Kids Exercising

"Train up a child in the way he should go; even when he is old, he will not depart from it."

— *Proverb 22:6.*

When engaging in the conversation of exercising, most people think of going to the gym, running on a treadmill, riding an exercise bike, or lifting weights, which is usually true.

But, when it comes to kids, exercise is not the same. For kids, exercise means anything that involves being active, like gym class, recess, riding their bikes, and so on.

Some of the benefits kids get from exercising include: developing stronger muscles and bones, having leaner bodies, having a lower chance of getting type-2 diabetes, having lower blood pressure and blood cholesterol levels, having a better attitude and outlook on life, and the ability to sleep better, and more.

Below are three elements of fitness that should be a part of kids' lives:

1. Endurance

Endurance develops when kids regularly get aerobic activity. This means the child is moving around, their hearts are beating faster, and breathing is labored. This strengthens the heart and improves the body's ability to send oxygen to all the cells of the body. Some activities include cycling, skating, swimming, tennis, walking, jogging, team sports, and more.

2. Strength

Strength does not have to mean lifting weights. Instead, kids can do push-ups, stomach crunches, pull-ups, and other exercises to help tone and strengthen muscles. They also improve their strength when they climb, do a handstand, wrestle, and more.

3. Flexibility

Stretching exercises, which tend to improve kids' muscles and joints, allow them to bend and move easily through their full range of motion, such as when they reach for a book, practice a split, or do a cartwheel.

The American Academy of Pediatrics (AAP) recommends:

- Parents limit their child's device time

- Keep TVs, computers, and video games out of children's bedrooms.

- Turn off screens during mealtimes.

It is suggested that kids, teens, and toddlers should get 60 minutes or more of moderate to vigorous physical activity daily.

Preschoolers should have at least 120 minutes of active play every day. Young children should not be inactive for hours on end. Typically, no more than 1 hour unless they're sleeping. And school-age children should not be inactive for periods longer than two hours.

How can we prevent or slow the onset of disease in kids? It is important to know that kids are not immune to diseases. Inactivity in kids leads to the same illnesses adults develop, including: hypertension, heart disease, various cancers, osteoporosis, depression, anxiety, obesity, and more.

Here are some tips for raising active kids:

• Have your kids do a variety of age-appropriate activities, especially if you have kids of multiple ages.

• Make being active a part of daily life, like taking the stairs instead of the elevator.

• Be a positive role model for your entire family and include group activities.

• And keep it fun, so you and your kids will want to do more.

And finally, add in a clean diet, and your children will be on the road to living a fit and healthy life they can pass on to their children and grandchildren.

Be Blessed!

Chapter 6 - Health Benefits Of Good Nutrition

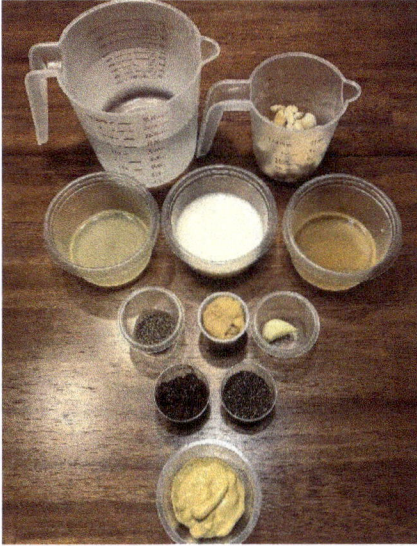

Healthy Diet Swaps

January 21st has been designated as World Swap Day. Originally started as a way to reinvent shopping, it's a movement that's gaining national attention and seeing activity across the country. World Swap Day encourages all to share goods, food, clothes, toys, or many other items versus buying them new. Swapping will turn any unused items into things you actually need. Therefore, you don't spend money, and you don't compile unused stuff around your house.

In celebration of World Swap Day, why not do some personal swapping for your health? Big results have come from small changes. For example, swapping fries for a medium baked potato saves you over 250 calories in your lunch, and you avoid all unhealthy oils. Swapping is easy and good for everybody.

Check out ten easy swaps you can do to celebrate World Swap Day and your health.

1. Swap your morning bacon for some baked Tempeh or tofu. You can season them and make them as flavorful as you like, and they contain much less fat.

2. Swap a soda for water with lemon. Even if it's just one soda, your body will thank you.

3. Swap a starch for a fresh vegetable. When preparing or ordering your sides, give up starch for a nutrient-rich vegetable. A favorite is swapping potatoes for steamed and mashed cauliflower!

4. Swap a sugary yogurt for Greek yogurt. Those deceiving cups labeled yogurt can be loaded with sugar and high fructose.com syrup, totally negating all the benefits of yogurt.

Opt for Greek yogurt. It is delicious and loaded with double the protein of a typical yogurt.

5. Swap meat for meatless. Get on board the Meatless Monday train, or make any day of the week meatless. This encourages more beans, lentils, vegetables, more fiber, and as a result, more nutrients and less fat in your recipes. There are tons of delicious and nutritious meatless meals – many so good you won't even notice the meat is missing.

6. Swap a drive-thru for the table. Even for a busy family, sitting down to eat isn't impossible. Check out crock-pot meals that simmer and cook all day while you work, and then they're ready to serve when you walk in the door. Also, keep wraps on hand. You can use leftovers, to make tasty wraps. Load the wrap-up and just add a healthy dressing of your choice. If you must eat out, try to stick to a place that doesn't have a drive-thru. Typically, if you have to sit in a restaurant, the food is healthier. Think Chipotle as an example.

7. Swap your "usual" for something new. Whether it's ordering a new menu item, using a new recipe, or picking out new produce, try something new. Never tried blood oranges? Give them a shot. Do you always have cereal for breakfast? Try an egg white omelet. Have fun with it. Let the kids pick out a new vegetable. Change is good.

Glycemic Index

Glycemic Index: What It Is and How to Use It

Genesis 1:29 Then God said:

"I give you every seed-bearing plant on the face of the whole earth and every tree that has fruit with seed in it. They will be yours for food…"

Just so you know, seed-bearing plants and fruit are LOW GI FOODS!

The glycemic index (Also known as GI) is a tool that's often used to promote better blood sugar management by measuring how much specific foods INCREASE blood sugar levels.

Several factors influence the glycemic index of a food, including its nutrient composition, cooking method, ripeness, and the amount of processing it has undergone.

The glycemic index can NOT only help increase your awareness of what you're putting on your plate but also enhance weight loss, decrease your blood sugar levels, and reduce both your HDL and LDL (the bad) cholesterol.

Foods are classified as low, medium, or high glycemic foods and ranked on a scale of 0–100.

The LOWER the GI of a specific food, the less it may affect your blood sugar levels (which is what we want)

The three GI ratings are:

- Low: 55 or less

- Medium: 56–69

- High: 70 or above

Foods high in refined carbs and sugar are digested more quickly and often have a high GI, which spikes blood sugar, while foods high in protein, fat, or fiber typically have a low GI. Foods that contain no carbs are not assigned a GI: THAT includes meat, fish, poultry, nuts, seeds, herbs, spices, and oils.

Keep in mind that the amount of food we eat does MATTER, even when we're eating healthy.

So some foods you can eat are:

- Fruits: such as apples, berries, oranges, lemons, limes, grapefruit

- Non-starchy vegetables: broccoli, cauliflower, carrots, spinach, tomatoes

- Whole grains: quinoa, couscous, barley, buckwheat, farro, oats

- Legumes: lentils, black beans, chickpeas and kidney beans

Foods without a GI value or with a very low GI can also be enjoyed IN VERY SMALL AMOUNTS...SUCH AS ON TOP OF A SALAD...as part of a balanced low GI (glycemic) diet. They include:

- Meat

- Seafood

- Poultry

- Nuts: almonds, macadamia nuts, walnuts, pistachios

- Seeds: chia seeds, sesame seeds, hemp seeds, flax seeds

- Herbs and spices: turmeric, black pepper, cumin, dill, basil, rosemary, cinnamon

Although no foods are strictly off-limits, foods with a HIGH GI should be limited, such as:

- Bread: white bread, bagels, naan, pita bread

- Rice: white rice, jasmine rice, arborio rice

- Cereals: instant oats, breakfast cereals

- Pasta and noodles: lasagna, spaghetti, ravioli, macaroni, fettuccine

- Starchy vegetables: mashed potatoes, potatoes, *french fries*

- Baked goods: cake, doughnuts, cookies, croissants, muffins

- Snacks: chocolate, crackers, *microwave popcorn*, chips, pretzels

- All Sugars [-sweetened beverages: soda, fruit juice, sports drinks, and things that include] especially HIGH FRUCTOSE CORN SYRUP

Ideally, try to replace these foods with foods that have a lower GI whenever possible.

You can search for a GI Food Chart on the internet and choose the best foods for you... as James and I always say, it's never too late to start TODAY!!!

Well, as always, I hope this has been a blessing to you. Pass it on to friends and family. And keep living fit and doing what matters.

Have a blessed day.

Clean Eating Pt. I

Tips on Eating Clean Pt. 1/3

Jeremiah 33:6 says:

"Nevertheless, I will bring health and healing to it; I will heal my people and will let them enjoy abundant peace and security."

Reading this passage lets us know that it's very obvious that God wants us to live an abundant life. How successful we are depends on our contribution. As in our spiritual lives, we must also put in the work when it comes to our physical lives!

We have evolved into nations that have adapted toxic eating habits. These habits have been socially accepted. As such, eating clean for most requires a lifestyle change, but it is a growing trend because more people realize the health benefits outweigh the effort it needs to change.

So here are two tips that will hopefully help you transition to a cleaner way of eating:

1. Eliminate Processed Foods

It's pretty easy to learn about the clean eating lifestyle, but following it can be complex and a significant shock to your body (but in a good way).

One of the main foundations of clean eating is cutting out and avoiding processed foods. Doing so will prevent the consumption of unhealthy and sometimes very harmful additives. Processed foods are hard on your body and have been connected to severe health complications, including cardiovascular disease and obesity. They can contain many harmful ingredients that are harmful to your liver and hard for you to digest, and those toxic ingredients and additives are often stored in the body.

Reading the ingredient list and nutritional information on the side of pre-made, packaged, and processed foods can be a real wake-up call if you haven't done so before. Processed foods can have an alarming amount of sodium, unhealthy fat, and sugar. To make it worse, after reading the label, you often realize that the serving size is only half or less of what you would typically eat. Next time you're shopping, skip processed foods to eat clean and significantly improve your health.

The second thing is, if possible...

2. Buy Local Foods

The simplest yet tricky aspect of clean eating is purchasing local foods. By buying locally, you cut out the food's travel time and possible packaging or processing. Unfortunately, even though buying local food is healthier for you and the environment and helps support local businesses, sometimes (NOT ALL), it's a bit more expensive than what you'll find at your local grocery store.

But [if you can afford it...] it's worth it and doesn't cost that much more in general—even less if you shop at farmer's markets, especially for fruits and vegetables, which are often cheaper from a local farm than a grocery store.

Although it's good to buy produce marked as from the state or province you live in, it's unlikely that what you buy is from the "actual" city you live in.

There's still some travel time and packaging involved; however, it's best to buy directly from the source as often as possible.

And that's it!

I pray this message has been beneficial and a blessing to you. Please pass it on to friends and family.

Be blessed!

Clean Eating Pt. II

Clean Eating Tips Part 2/3

1st Corinthians 10:13 says:

"No temptation has overtaken you except what is common to mankind. And God is faithful; he will not let you be tempted beyond what you can bear. But when you are tempted, he will also provide a way out so that you can endure it."

As I said previously, God wants us to be healthy and live an abundant life. He gave us free will, and we can use that will to make good or bad food choices. Whatever we choose, like in all things, there will be consequences.

More and more people are becoming aware of the benefits of eating clean, changing their lifestyles, and buying locally.

Clean eating changes how you eat, how much, and when you eat. It encourages altering your diet and removing processed foods to eat fresh produce and whole grains packed full of nutrients and other foods that contain good fats to improve overall health.

This lifestyle has many health benefits, including reducing the risk of cardiovascular disease, many types of cancers, and other medical problems.

Awareness of your food's journey from the garden to your plate removes additives, fillers, and other unnecessary products.

Here are two more tips to help you transition to a cleaner way of eating:

1. Eat Several Small Meals a Day

Many people who follow a clean lifestyle eat several small meals daily. If you typically eat 1-3 big meals/day, you may want to change that to 4- 6 smaller meals instead.

Some benefits of eating this way include improving metabolism and maintaining blood sugar levels. It can also prevent overeating because you won't feel starving at your next meal; plus, It provides your body with a regular source of nourishment to keep you energized and satiated throughout the day.

Do not eat…Processed foods because they often leave you undernourished, still hungry, and scouring for more food and snacks to fill the void.

Be sure to include foods high in fiber (including plenty of fruits and vegetables) so you don't feel hungry throughout the day.

AND...

2. Exercise Portion Control

Even if you're an exercise junkie or are training for a physically demanding activity, portion control is an essential aspect of clean eating that's doable regardless of your situation.

Everyone requires different amounts of food, depending on their age, sex, weight, medical history, and lifestyle. Through portion control, you can still get the added protein you need to train while loading up on vital nutrients that will help your overall health.

I pray that this message has been a blessing to you. Share this information with friends and family.

Be blessed!

Clean Eating Pt. III

Proverbs 16:19 says:

"Better to live humbly with the poor then to share plunder with the proud."

Once again, God wants us to be healthy and live an abundant life. However, it is up to us to make the right choices.

More and more people are becoming aware of the benefits of eating clean, changing their lifestyles, buying local, and staying away from processed foods.

Clean eating changes how you eat, how much, and when you eat. It encourages you to eat fresh produce and whole grains packed with nutrients to improve overall health.

The health benefits of this lifestyle are numerous, including reducing the risk of obesity, cardiovascular disease, many types of cancers, and other medical problems.

Being aware of the nature of the food we eat allows us to control the kind of nourishment or lack thereof we provide our bodies with.

At this point, we know that to eat clean, we must:

1. Eliminate processed foods

2. Buy Local

3. Eat several small meals and,

4. Exercise portion control

Here are the last two tips in this three-part series that will hopefully help you transition to a cleaner way of eating:

1. Drink Water

Clean eating is about keeping your body clean in every aspect, allowing it to flourish, and helping your body become as healthy and strong as possible.

Water is vital for your body and impacts more of your health than you may know. It can flush out toxins and other harmful waste in the body, enhance and maintain healthy muscles, and decrease joint pain.

Some teas and other fluids can be as effective in hydrating your body as water, so if drinking a lot of water is a significant challenge to you, you could supplement a few cups of herbal tea as your body and mind adjust to the change.

Staying hydrated is also known to help control your appetite. Hunger is often mistaken for thirst, causing people to eat and overeat instead of giving the body what it needs: water.

You should drink a minimum of 8 8-ounce servings of water a day or more, based on how active you are.

And the final tip for eating clean is...

2. One of the most important, in my opinion, shop the perimeter of the store (the outer sides):

Consider how grocery stores are typically laid out, and you'll notice how most items are in boxes, jars, and other packages; think further about it, and you'll realize how those inner aisles and shelves contain pre-made, frozen, and, ultimately, heavily processed foods!

You'll avoid the worst processed foods by shopping the perimeter of your grocery store.

It's not a perfect answer to clean eating since produce, meats, and dairy found in grocery stores are often imported from other countries, but it limits unhealthy food choices and drastically reduces the number of hidden sugar purchases. And that will positively impact your diet and overall health. And, of course, you can contribute to your local farmers and community by buying local products as often as possible.

I pray that this message has been a blessing to you. Share this information with friends and family.

Be blessed!

Night/Binge Eating

Courtesy of the GREEN MOUNTAIN at Fox RUN in Vermont:

A Weight Loss Retreat.

1st Corinthians 10:31 says:

"So whether you eat or drink or whatever you do, do it all for the glory of God."

When we are not seeing the physical results we want from our eating habits, we have to examine our eating habits.

Do you restrict how much food you eat? Do you deprive yourself or skip meals throughout the day?

And as a result, are you thinking about food all the time?

What about this scenario:

You go all day without eating; you have not prepared anything for dinner, so you grab take-out. And, after you've eaten, you munch on snacks on and off throughout the night.

Then you justify it by saying, "I haven't eaten all day, so I deserve it!"

So now... you feel guilty, not just because you know better, but because you haven't done better.

Does this sound familiar to you???

The reality is... we should be eating to glorify God. Not aimless eating and gouging ourselves just for the satisfaction or taste of it.

If this scenario fits you, you are a night/binge eater.

And studies show...you're not alone. According to the National Institute of Mental Health, over 1.5% of the US population (over five million people) deals with this issue.

And as a result, you end up setting yourself up for numerous illnesses.

Intentionally not eating almost always leads to overeating or binging. Because we begin to feel deprived, and thus, we attempt to make up for what we missed.

So, Here are a few tips I hope will help you... to STOP EATING AT NIGHT!

Eat more food during the day! MAKE SURE IT'S Nutritious foods,

1. Try eating whole grain oats, grits, or a large smoothie in the morning, then later, with Lt. dressing, fruits, or

unsalted nuts and seeds, and drink plenty of water throughout the day...This will keep you feeling full longer.

2. Switch up your nightly routine:

3. If you snack while watching TV, try reading a book or plan something to do during the commercial, like folding laundry or putting the dishes away.

4. If you snack while surfing the web or on social media, try logging off for a few hours or a few days. When you log back on, you'll realize you didn't miss anything that important.

5. Finally, try going to bed a little earlier. I do this all the time. Chances are, you will avoid mindless eating by calling it a night earlier. If you should wake up in the middle of the night, try to have a low-fat snack available, like a banana or apple, so you will feel satisfied enough to go back to bed after you brush your teeth.

Keep in mind that it will take at least 30 days to develop a new habit, so do not give up if you don't get it right on the first try.

Have a blessed day!

Now, to move away from personal behaviors to specific foods and their nutritional benefits.

Celery

Ecclesiastes 9:7 says:

"Go, eat your food with gladness, and drink your wine with a joyful heart, for God has already approved what you do."

Celery was initially used as a medicinal herb. It was used for:

- Treating arthritis and gout

- Helping reduce muscle spasms

- Calming the nerves

- Reducing inflammation

- Lowering blood pressure...and more

Celery is now a common ingredient in kitchens worldwide.

The stalks are rich in cellulose, a complex carbohydrate found in the cell wall of plants that is edible (but indigestible to humans, which makes it a catalyst to move toxins out of the body).

Most people think celery has no nutritional value because of its high water content of 95%. However, the remaining 5% contains some of the most powerful micronutrients found in any vegetable, making it a valuable health food and addition to any meal.

According to the USDA: 1 medium (7 1/2" to 8" long) celery stalk (40g).[1]

- **Calories**: 5.6

- **Fat**: 0.1g

- **Sodium**: 32mg

- **Carbohydrates**: 1.2g

- **Fiber**: 0.6g

- **Sugars**: 0.5g and even

- **Protein**: 0.3g

Making it a popular choice on **low-calorie diets**.

Despite its low-calorie content, Celery contains micronutrients…Such as **potassium, folate, choline, vitamin A,** and **vitamin K**. Celery also provides some natural **sodium** and fluoride.

The Health Benefits of celery are numerous; it has a profound impact on- Diabetes Prevention and Wellness Management.

The **flavonoids** in celery are protective against oxidative damage to the beta cells of the pancreas. These cells are responsible for producing insulin and regulating glucose levels. They also stop the progression of diabetes by preventing cataracts, retinopathy (blindness), and neuropathy (decreased sensations in hands and feet). Celery is also high in quercetin, a powerful antioxidant that increases glucose uptake in the liver and stimulates insulin secretion to help keep diabetes from progressing.

It also lowers blood pressure, reduces cholesterol levels, and prevents inflammation.

Although celery provides some natural sodium, it is high in polyphenols that are anti-inflammatory and protective against cardiovascular disease.

You can purchase Celery in practically any store.

Celery stalks are best when they are crisp and green. They should be free from signs of dryness, brown spots, cracks, or limpness.

Although most people discard celery leaves, they ARE edible and can make a good addition to soup, pesto, and smoothies. Chopped celery leaves (work) great on salads, sandwiches, and cooked dishes.

Raw or cooked, you can place them in side dishes like stuffing. Dip celery into peanut butter, hummus, yogurt dip, tuna, or chicken salad. Celery's natural crunch and salty flavor makes it a healthy substitute for chips or crackers.

And there you have it!!!

I pray this message has been a blessing to you; please pass it on to family and friends and be blessed.

Berries

One of the Healthiest Foods on Earth

I'm going to share three reasons why I feel you should add berries to your diet!

First of all, please check with your doctor before consuming berries, especially if you are allergic to them or are on a low-fiber diet.

1. The first reason I feel you should add berries to your diet is that berries are loaded with antioxidants, which help keep free radicals under control. Free radicals are unstable molecules beneficial in small amounts but can damage your cells when their numbers get too high, causing oxidative stress.

In addition to protecting your cells, berry plant compounds may reduce the risk of disease.

One study shows that blackberries, blueberries, and raspberries have the highest antioxidant activity of commonly consumed fruits, even in as little as a 10oz portion.

2. The second reason you should add berries to your diet comes from a study that SHOWS how berries may improve your blood sugar and insulin levels.

They even reduce blood sugar and insulin response after eating a high-carb meal.

In the study, women were given 5 oz of pureed strawberries or mixed berries with bread. They had a 24 to 26% reduction in insulin levels compared to consuming the bread alone.

3. You should add berries to your diet because they are high in fiber, including soluble fiber. Studies show that consuming soluble fiber slows down the movement of food through your digestive tract, leading to reduced hunger and increased feelings of fullness.

This is awesome for weight management. Because it may decrease your caloric intake, helping you to lose weight better. One study found that doubling your fiber intake could make you absorb up to 130 fewer calories daily.

A typical serving size for berries is one cup:

(which converts to about 4.4 to 5.3 oz depending on the berry type)

There are organic and wild berries available worldwide now, and when they're not in season, you can freeze them or buy them frozen and thaw them as needed, and they can be enjoyed in almost every type of diet, food, and smoothie.

Although baked berries are considered processed, the total antioxidant concentrations remain the same and positively affect the arteries in people who consume baked or freeze-dried berries.

So the bottom line on berries is they taste great, are highly nutritious, and provide many health benefits, including for your heart and skin. So, by including them in your diet regularly, you can delightfully improve your overall health.

3 John 1:2 says:

"Dear friend, I hope all is well with you and that you are as healthy in body as you are strong in spirit."

Remember that God wants us to be spiritually and physically healthy so he can use our vessels to spread the gospel!

I pray that this message has been a blessing to you and helps you remain steadfast and deeply rooted as you continue your walk with Christ and live a healthy lifestyle.

Evidence-Based Health Benefits of Magnesium

Psalms 145:15 says:

"The eyes of all look to you, and you give them their food at the proper time."

From regulating blood sugar levels to boosting athletic performance, magnesium is crucial for your brain and body.

Yet, although it's found in a variety of foods ranging from leafy greens to nuts, seeds, and beans, many people don't get enough in their diet.

Here are four things I feel you should know about Magnesium:

First, It's Involved in hundreds of biochemical reactions in your body. Magnesium is found throughout your body. In fact, every cell in your body contains this mineral and needs it to function. About 60% of the magnesium in your body occurs in bone, while the rest is in muscles, soft tissues, and fluids, including blood.

One of its main roles is to act as a cofactor — a helper molecule — in the biochemical reactions continuously performed by enzymes. It's involved in more than 600 reactions in your body, including:

-Energy creation: converting food into energy.

-Protein formation: creating new proteins from **amino acids.**

-Gene maintenance: helping create and repair DNA and RNA.

-Muscle movements: aiding in muscle contraction and relaxation.

-Nervous system regulation: regulating neurotransmitters, which send messages throughout your brain and nervous system.

Nonetheless, studies suggest that approximately 50% of U.S. adults get less than the recommended daily amount of magnesium.

Second, Magnesium may boost exercise performance. During exercise, you need more magnesium than when you're resting, depending on the activity. Studies show magnesium helps move blood sugar into your muscles and dispose of lactate, which can build up during exercise and cause fatigue. Studies also suggest that magnesium supplements protect against certain markers of muscle damage in professional cyclists.

Third, magnesium may combat depression. Magnesium plays a critical role in brain function and mood, and low levels are linked to an increased risk of depression.

In fact, an analysis of data from more than 8,800 people found that those under age 65 with the lowest magnesium intake had a 22% greater risk of depression... and

Fourth, magnesium boasts anti-inflammatory benefits and more. Low magnesium intake is linked to increased levels of inflammation, which plays a key role in aging and chronic disease.

One review of 11 studies concluded that magnesium supplements decreased levels of C-reactive protein (CRP), a marker of inflammation, in people with chronic inflammation. Other studies report similar findings, showing that magnesium supplements may reduce CRP and other markers of inflammation.

The good news is that much of the poor effects of having low levels of this mineral can be reversed, or even eliminated, by taking supplements or eating foods rich in magnesium, such as...

Pumpkin seeds: 37% of the DV per ounce (28 grams)

Chia seeds: 26% of the DV per ounce (28 grams)

Spinach boiled: 19% of the DV per 1/2 cup (90 grams)

Almonds: 19% of the DV per ounce (28 grams)

Cashews: 18% of the DV per ounce (28 grams)

Black beans cooked: 14% of the DV per 1/2 cup (86 grams)

Edamame, cooked: 12% of the DV per 1/2 cup (78 grams)

Peanut butter: 12% of the DV per 2 tablespoons (32 grams)

Brown rice, cooked: 10% of the DV per 1/2 cup (100 grams)

Salmon, cooked: 6% of the DV per 3 ounces (85 grams)

Halibut cooked: 6% of the DV per 3 ounces (85 grams)

Avocado: 5% of the DV per 1/2 cup (75 grams)

As for supplements:

If you have a medical condition, check with your doctor before taking magnesium supplements. Though supplements are generally well tolerated, they may be unsafe for people who take certain diuretics, heart medications, or antibiotics. So definitely check with your doctor.

The bottom line is Magnesium is essential for maintaining good health!

I pray this message has been a blessing to you. Please pass it on to family and friends, and be blessed!

Ways to control high blood pressure without medications

Choosing a healthy lifestyle is "Key" to living disease-free. When James and I go to a hotel, we make sure we straighten up the room before we leave. Knowing that it is not our property, we take measures to take care of it. And we should live our lives the same way, knowing that these bodies are not our own.

1 Corinthians 6:19-20 says:

"What? know ye not that your body is the temple of the Holy Ghost which is in you, which ye have of God, and ye are not your own?"

By making lifestyle changes, you can lower your blood pressure and reduce your risk of heart disease. Here are just four examples of what you can do, courtesy of the Mayo Clinic:

1.   Lose extra pounds and watch your waistline

Blood pressure often increases as weight increases. Being overweight also can cause disrupted breathing while you sleep (sleep apnea), which further raises blood pressure.

Weight loss is one of the most effective lifestyle changes for controlling blood pressure and many other diseases. If you're overweight, losing even a small amount of weight can help reduce blood pressure. Having a normal BMI (body weight based on height) is one of the best things you can do to prevent diseases.

[- In general, blood pressure might go down by about "1 millimeter of mercury" (mm Hg) with each kilogram (about 2.2 pounds) of weight lost.-]

Also, the size of the waistline is important. Carrying too much weight around the waist can increase the risk of high blood pressure.

Typically:

Men are at risk if their waist measurement is greater than 40 inches (102 centimeters).

Women are at risk if their waist measurement is greater than 35 inches (89 centimeters).

2. Get regular exercise:

Regular physical activity can lower high blood pressure.

[by about 5 to 8 mm Hg.]

It's important to exercise to keep blood pressure from rising. As a general goal, aim for at least 30 minutes of moderate physical activity every day. You don't have to be extreme or try to break Olympic records. Just be consistent.

Exercise can also help keep elevated blood pressure from turning into high blood pressure (known as hypertension). For those who have hypertension, regular physical activity can bring blood pressure down to safer levels.

Some examples of aerobic exercise that can help lower blood pressure include walking, jogging, cycling, swimming, and dancing. Also, high-intensity interval training (HIIT) and strength training can help reduce blood pressure.

3.   Decrease the amount of salt (sodium) in your diet.

Even a small reduction of sodium in the diet can improve heart health and reduce high blood pressure (by about 5 to 6 mm Hg).

The effect of sodium intake on blood pressure varies among groups of people.

Most people are taking in about 3,200 mg of sodium per day. The CDC says 2,500 is the amount at which health problems begin to arise. They recommend 2,300 milligrams (mg) a day, which is ideal for good health and even less if you're over the age of 50.

To reduce sodium in the diet:

Read food labels. Look for low-sodium versions of foods and beverages.

Eat fewer processed foods. Only a small amount of sodium occurs naturally in foods. Most sodium is added during processing. Processed foods come from eating out, and many packaged foods are bought at grocery stores.

Don't add salt. Use herbs or spices to add flavor to food.

Cook your own food!!! Cooking lets you control the amount of sodium and seasonings, in general, in your food.

And,

4. Get adequate rest/sleep

Studies show poor sleep quality — i.e. getting fewer than six hours of sleep every night for several weeks — can contribute to hypertension. Any number of issues can disrupt sleep.

Try to:

-   Stick to a sleep schedule. Go to bed and wake up at the same time each day. Try to keep the same schedule on weeknights and on weekends.

-   Create a restful space. That means keeping the sleeping space cool, quiet, and dark. Do something relaxing in the hour before bedtime. That might include taking a warm bath or doing relaxation exercises. Avoid bright light, such as from a TV or computer screen.

-    Watch what you eat and drink. Don't go to bed hungry or stuffed. Avoid large meals close to bedtime. Limit or avoid nicotine, caffeine, and alcohol close to bedtime, as well…and finally:

-    Limit naps. For those who find napping during the day helpful, limiting naps to 30 minutes earlier in the day might help nighttime sleep.

I pray this message has been a blessing to you. Please pass it on to family and friends.

Be blessed!

The Health Benefits of Curcumin and Turmeric

This section will give you some scientifically proven health benefits of turmeric and curcumin:

Revelation 22:2:

"Amid the street of it, and on either side of the river, [was there] the tree of life, which bare twelve [manner of] fruits, [and] yielded her fruit every month: and the leaves of the tree [were] for the healing of the nations."

Turmeric is a spice with a long history of use as a traditional medicine. It is a potent, flavorful spice primarily cultivated in parts of Southeast Asia. Aside from giving Curry its vibrant yellow color, turmeric is also known for its many health benefits.

Curcumin is the primary active component of turmeric and the one that gives the spice its characteristically yellow color.

Unfortunately, turmeric and curcumin (Together or individually) don't absorb well into the bloodstream. To reach health benefits, researchers claim you need to add black pepper to the turmeric and curcumin...

A black pepper compound called Piperine helps make the turmeric bioavailable once ingested. In other words, black pepper increases the absorbability of turmeric and curcumin and how much they can use. Studies show that 20 mg of piperine and two grams of curcumin increase bioactivity(absorption) by 2,000 percent.

So, the following are some of the many health benefits of using turmeric and curcumin as part of a healthy diet:

1. Curcumin is an anti-inflammatory agent, meaning it treats conditions like bowel disease, pancreatitis, and arthritis

2. Curcumin may protect against heart disease and Osteo and Rheumatoid Arthritis; studies show that due to its anti-inflammatory agents, curcumin May improve the endothelial function or the health of the thin membrane that covers the inside of the heart and blood vessels, which plays a massive role in regulating blood pressure.

3. Curcumin may prevent cancer... curcumin is widely known as an anti-inflammatory compound that plays a huge role in treating and preventing a variety of cancers, including colorectal pancreas, prostate, breast, and gastric.

4. Studies also show that turmeric helps in the treatment and prevention of diabetes:

For example, studies showed that animals were fed 80 mg per 1g of body wt. of tetra-hydro curcumin, one of the main substances, and curcumin... And found that there was a significant decrease in blood sugar as well as an increase in plasma insulin.

5. Turmeric has also been found to help delay or reverse Alzheimer's disease and DEPRESSION.

6. Turmeric improves skin health, works as an anti-aging supplement, and prevents eye degeneration.

7. And finally, turmeric protects your body from free radicals, which are known to damage the fats and proteins in your system and even your DNA, which could lead to many of the diseases I mentioned earlier. Curcumin scavenges the different types of free radicals and controls and neutralizes them, preventing them from causing damage to the body.

These excellent spices come in pill form and powder. It's available in shaker form to bulk size, with a price range from a few dollars and higher. They can be found in most grocery stores, health food stores, and Asian and international stores.

So remember, one of your primary goals should be to do everything you can to stay fit and healthy, and adding turmeric with curcumin is a great way to help you achieve that goal.

I pray that this message has blessed you or someone you know. Please feel free to pass this information on to your friends and family.

Be blessed!

Veganuary!

Here is another tool to add to your healthy eating regimen.

Bible Verse: 3 JOHN 1:2:

"Beloved, I wish above all things that thou mayest prosper and be in health even as thy Soul prospereth."

Are you someone who has chronic illnesses? Or do you know someone who does? If so, here is a great opportunity to take steps to reverse it. January is also known as Veganuary!

January marks a time of the year when we reassess everything we do, from spiritual to exercising to career choices... and more.

As part of this self-assessment, one of the things people look at is their diet and what changes they may want to make. Veganuary began as a challenge for people to take a pledge to give up meat, dairy, and eggs during January.

This is an opportunity to make significant changes that could benefit not just your health but also animal welfare and the environment (or your carbon footprint).

There are many studies showing evidence that a whole food vegan diet can reduce your risk of chronic diseases like type 2 diabetes, 13 different types of cancer, heart disease, and stroke, and reduce blood pressure.

A recent study by Oxford University found going vegan can reduce your carbon footprint by up to 73%, largely because producing plant-based foods requires significantly less farmland than meat and dairy production.

So how do you get started? Start by keeping staple items in your pantry, such as quinoa, which is a complete protein, oatmeal, nutritional yeast, and plant-based milk, which provides calcium and other important nutrients. These are items you can use every day and in a variety of recipes.

50,000 people took the challenge in 2020, and a whopping 72% of them said they would continue with a vegan diet after the month was over.

20 years ago, vegan foods were mainly sold in speciality stores, but today, they are everywhere! Most stores and restaurants offer vegan foods of all kinds. Plus, you can order online, google recipes and buy countless cookbooks to help get started. And there's a fantastic event going around the country called Vegan Fest, which has gained momentum over the years. I suggest you can do an online search for an event in your area. You can bring the whole family, and I think you will enjoy it!

So, if you are looking for another opportunity to improve your health, try going vegan for a while.

Be Blessed!

Chapter 7 - Recipes

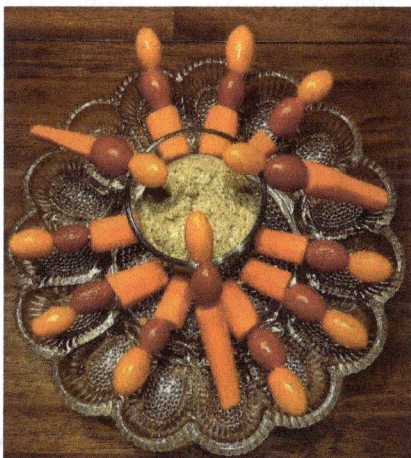

Smoothies

Awesome Healthy Green Smoothie

1 Corinthians 10:31:

"So whether you eat or drink, or whatever you do, do it all for the glory of God."

(and this is why we want to stay healthy)

Now, For this recipe, all you need are five ingredients:

All organic, if possible, to avoid herbicides and pesticides. But, If not possible, just wash everything carefully.

- 6 oz. spinach
- 2 stalks of chopped celery
- 1-2 med.-lg. orange(s)
- 1-2 cup(s) chopped pineapple and
- 1 med.-lg. banana

(SPINACH, an ORANGE or two, a PINEAPPLE, and a BANANA)

Nutritional Value of ingredients:

Spinach - Spinach has an extremely high nutritional value and is rich in antioxidants. It is a good source of vitamins A, B2, C, and K and also contains magnesium, manganese, folate, iron, calcium, potassium, and flavonoids, which are known to help the body protect from lung and oral cavity cancers.

Calories 39, Fat .66g, Carbs. 6.17g, Protein 4.86

Celery - Celery's health benefits are numerous, including lowering inflammation, reducing cholesterol, treating high blood pressure, aiding in weight loss, fighting infection, reducing the risk of urinary tract infection, improving mood, helping sleep, fighting cramps, keeping cancer at bay, boosting the immune system, improves eye health, boosts energy and brain health and reduces blood sugar levels.

Calories 17, Fat .21g, Carbs. 3.68, Protein .86g

Orange - You may need two because you'll need to squeeze out a whole cup., whole fruit is better because you get more fiber: Frozen is okay - 1 cup (juice):

Oranges are low in calories. They contain no saturated fats or cholesterol but are rich in dietary fiber, and pectin.

Calories 62, Fat .16g, Carbs. 15.39g, Protein 1.23g

Pineapple - (Frozen preferably) 1 cup pineapple is loaded with nutrients. They contain disease-fighting antioxidants. Its enzymes can ease digestion and may help reduce cancer risk. They provide a high supply of vitamin C, vitamin B1, potassium, and manganese, in addition to other special antioxidants that help prevent disease.

Calories 74, Fat .19g, Carbs. 19.58, Protein .84g

Banana - (Preferably ripe, peeled, and if possible frozen): Bananas are one of the most popular fruits on earth, and for a good reason. They are a great dietary source of potassium. A potassium-rich diet can help lower blood pressure, and people who eat plenty of potassium have up to a 27% lower risk of heart disease. Bananas also help with reducing obesity, arthritis, gout, kidney and urinary disorders, menstrual problems, and get this, burns. Banana peels and leaves are antibiotics. Another good reason to use banana leaves and peels for burns and wounds is that they are antimicrobial. Yes, they inhibit the growth of bacteria or fungal infections that can seriously interfere with the healing of a burn or wound.

Calories 89, Fat .3g, Carbs. 22.8g, Protein 1.1g

Okay, so there are all of your ingredients. Now, here's all you do.

Put all of the ingredients in a blender (A hi-speed is best, but a regular blender will work also) and blend to the consistency you desire. Blending these ingredients makes the nutrients more absorbable than eating them. Separately, Pour and enjoy!

You can use add-ons and make substitutions such as:

• Any leafy greens

• Most Frozen fruits are okay: peaches, mango, blueberries, apples, etc.

• And avocado

This recipe yields three servings of fruits and three vegetables in each cup… It's about 300 calories!

Thanks, and be blessed!!!

Oatmeal With Fruit, Nuts, And Seeds

Serves 4 cups.

Ingredients:

- 1 cup old-fashioned or steel-cut oats.

- 2 cups water.

- Pinch of salt and pepper.

- Almond or soy milk.

- Optional toppings: Honey (or maple syrup), walnuts, pumpkin seeds, banana, mixed berries, chia seeds, flaxseeds.

Instructions:

In a pot, combine oats, water, salt, and pepper. Bring to a boil, then reduce heat to a low simmer.

Partially cover and cook as directed on the package. Stirring occasionally to prevent it from sticking to the bottom of the pot.

Remove from heat and add milk and toppings to taste!

Oatmeal tips:

1.   To shorten cooking time, soak oats in water overnight in the fridge. In the morning, they'll take only about 10 - 15 minutes to cook!

2.   Let the oats simmer for about ten minutes, then turn off the heat and leave them covered on the stove for an hour while working out or doing a morning activity. When you return, the water is absorbed, and the oats are ready to eat!

3.   The oatmeal will keep covered in the fridge for up to 4 days. Gently rewarm before serving, and stir in a little extra almond milk or water to loosen it up.

Nutritional Value of the Ingredients:

Oats - Oats are incredibly nutritious. They are a great source of carbs and a powerful fiber called beta-glucan. They also contain high-quality protein, which provides a balance of essential amino acids to the body, important minerals, antioxidant plant compounds, and vitamins, such as the following:

Manganese: 63.91% of the daily value (DV)

Phosphorus: 13.3% of the DV

Magnesium: 13.3% of the DV

Copper: 17.6% of the DV

Iron: 9.4% of the DV

Zinc: 13.4% of the DV

Folate: 3.24% of the DV

Vitamin B1 (thiamin): 15.5% of the DV

Vitamin B5 (pantothenic acid): 9.07% of the DV

smaller amounts of calcium, potassium, vitamin B6 (pyridoxine), and vitamin B3 (niacin)

Oats are high in antioxidants, most notably avenanthramides, and beneficial plant compounds called polyphenols. Avenanthramides have anti-inflammatory and anti-itching effects. They help to lower blood pressure by increasing the production of nitric oxide, a gas molecule that helps open the blood vessels, leading to better blood flow.

The beta-glucan I mentioned previously is a soluble fiber that dissolves in water and makes a thick, gel-like substance in the gut, and as a result, helps reduce the LDL and total cholesterol, blood sugar, and insulin levels in respect. It also increases the amount of good bacteria in the gut and promotes feelings of fullness, diminishing feelings of hunger. Good news, especially for people trying to lose weight.

All in all, oats are among the nutrient-dense foods you can eat.

Rolled Oats: Calories: (½ cup) Calories 140, Carbs 28g, Protein 5g, Fat: 2.5g.

Steel Cut Oats: Calories: 603, Carbs 29g, Protein 7g, Fat 3g.

Milk (¼ cup) - Almond milk is light in flavor and a non-dairy, nutritious, nut-based alternative to cow's milk.

You can make almond milk by soaking, grinding, and straining raw almonds. Commercial versions of almond milk might add nutrients, such as calcium, riboflavin, vitamin E, and vitamin D, to boost the drink's nutritional content. And many people drink it just because they like the taste.

Almond Milk: Calories: 10, Protein 38g, Carbs: 35g, Fat: .09g.

Soy Milk: Calories: 32, Fat: .9g, Carbs: .35g, Protein: .38g.

Honey (Maple Syrup) (1 tbsp.) - Honey is a syrupy liquid that honeybees make from plant nectar. It is a common ingredient in many foods and is available in many forms. Honey is rich in nutrients and antioxidants, has antibacterial properties, and can play a role in diabetes management as part of a balanced diet. It also plays a role in many home remedies and alternative medicine treatments.

Honey is essentially pure sugar, with no fat and only trace amounts of protein and fiber. Also, it is worth noting that honey is rich in health-promoting plant compounds known as polyphenols. Darker varieties tend to offer more antioxidants than lighter varieties.

Although there are not a lot of studies on honey available, Studies show honey is beneficial for heart health, including reduced blood pressure and blood fat levels.

However, remember that honey is a type of sugar, so consuming it will cause your blood sugar levels to rise. Eating large quantities of honey, especially consistently over a long period, can contribute to weight gain and increase your risk of diseases like type 2 diabetes or heart disease. So limit your intake.

Calories: 1 tbsp. 60, Fat 0, Protein 0, Carbs 17g.

Walnuts (1 tbsp.) - Walnuts are packed with nutrients. They contain omega-3 fats, higher amounts of antioxidants than most foods, and other compounds that may help protect against brain decline, heart disease, and cancer. They originated in the Mediterranean region and Central Asia and have been part of the human diet for thousands of years.

Literature shows that eating walnuts may improve brain health and prevent heart disease and cancer. Walnuts are most often eaten on their own as a snack and added to baked goods. Walnuts are made up of 65% fat and about 15% of protein. They're low in carbs — most of which consist of fiber.

Like other nuts, most of the calories in walnuts come from fat. This makes them energy-dense, high-calorie food.

Even though walnuts are rich in fat and calories, studies indicate that they don't increase obesity risk when replacing other foods in your diet.

Walnuts are also richer than most other nuts in polyunsaturated fats. The most abundant one is an omega-6 fatty acid called linoleic acid.

They also contain a relatively high percentage of healthy omega-3 alpha-linolenic acid (ALA). This makes up around 8–14% of the total fat content. As such, walnuts are the only nuts that contain significant amounts of ALA. ALA helps reduce inflammation and improve the composition of blood fats, making it a heart-healthy food.

Calories: 67, Carbs 0g, Fat 6.6g, Protein 1.6g.

Pumpkin Seeds (1 tbsp) - Pumpkin seeds are a calorie-dense snack with several vitamins and minerals and are a very satisfying food. This tiny seed offers huge health benefits, including magnesium, zinc, and protein, along with protection against cancers, improved sleep, boosts heart health, eases menopausal symptoms, and helps with digestion.

Also, It is possible to have an allergic reaction to pumpkin seeds, although reports of this allergy are very rare. Allergies can develop at any time. Pumpkin meat or seed allergy symptoms may include chest tightness, hives, and vomiting. If you suspect an allergy to pumpkin, seek care from a healthcare professional.

Calories: 65, Fat 4.9g, Carbs 1.1g, Protein 3g.

Banana (1 med.) - One medium banana contains around 3g of fiber.1 That fiber can be broken down into two key parts: soluble and insoluble fiber.

Soluble fiber absorbs water to form a kind of gel. This gel slows digestion, allowing foods to be processed properly. This also allows sugar to be released more slowly. Some soluble fiber is made up of resistant starches that don't get digested and therefore end up in the large intestine as *prebiotics*. That means they're ready to feed the friendly bacteria in your gut.

Insoluble fiber adds bulk to stools. It helps to move waste through the digestive system (to avoid constipation). It also works to make you feel fuller while supporting healthy cholesterol.

Bananas will change from green to yellow once picked and will show brown spots when ripe. You may have heard people recommend eating slightly green, unripe bananas. This is because bananas have most of these two fibers before they're completely ripe. As they ripen, these fibers start to decrease slowly. In addition, green bananas have less sugar, making them a bit healthier for you.

Aside from aiding digestive health, bananas are filled with vitamins and minerals. These include:

Potassium - acts as a natural electrolyte. Electrolytes help maintain a balance of water in the cells and an electrical charge. This charge sparks cell function in the body, such as helping the muscle contractions that keep your heart beating.

Bananas are one of the most potassium-rich foods. The potassium content of bananas can also help to offset sodium in the body, supporting healthy blood pressure levels. Bananas are also a great natural remedy for leg muscle cramps because of their high potassium level.

Vitamin B6 - is required for more than 100 enzyme reactions involving metabolism. Research has shown that those with low levels of vitamin B6 may have double the risk of experiencing a heart issue.

Magnesium - helps keep nerve and muscle function in check. It also supports healthy bones and blood pressure and is needed to produce energy.

Vitamin C - aids the growth and repair process of body tissue by supporting skin health. This vitamin also helps maintain your cartilage, bones, and teeth. As a key antioxidant,

Vitamin C also fights free radicals that can prematurely age your skin and body.

Manganese - plays a role in the metabolism of carbohydrates, amino acids, and cholesterol. It's also essential for bone and skeletal development.

As far as carbs go, bananas are not comparable to processed junk food or refined grains. The positives of eating bananas should far outweigh any carb concerns.

Calories: 105, Fat 39, Carbs:26.95, Protein:1.29.

Mixed berries (1/2 cup) - Berries are one of the most versatile little foods you can eat. They are available everywhere. There are dozens of varieties of berries.

Berries have been classified as "superfoods" because they pack a lot of nutritional power into a tiny package. They are rich in antioxidants, which can prevent cell damage and may reduce the risk of certain diseases, including eye, heart, and kidney disease, high blood pressure, spikes in blood sugar, and cancer. The antioxidants found in berries are responsible for many of their health-boosting properties.

Berries are also high in fiber, which can help lower your cholesterol. Soluble fiber "catches" harmful cholesterol as it passes through your intestines, carrying it out as waste.

Research shows that this may reduce harmful cholesterol in your blood and help protect your heart.

Since there are many different kinds of berries, I will give you the nutritional value of blueberries and blackberries:

A half-cup serving of blueberries contains:

Calories: 42

Protein: 1 gram

Carbohydrates: 11 grams

Fiber: 2 grams

Sugar: 7 grams

Vitamin C: 7 milligrams

A half-cup serving of blackberries has a slightly different nutritional content:

Calories: 31

Protein: 1 gram

Carbohydrates: 7 grams

Fiber: 4 grams

Sugar: 3 grams

Vitamin C: 15 milligrams

Chia Seeds (1 tsp.) – Chia seeds are the tiny black (brown or white) seeds of the chia plant. Chia seeds contain large amounts of fiber and omega-3 fatty acids, plenty of protein, and many essential minerals and antioxidants. They may help improve digestive health, lower blood pressure, and improve blood sugar control.

Chia seeds contain 138 calories per ounce (28 grams). By weight, they are 6% water, 46% carbohydrates (of which 83% is fiber), 34% fat, and 19% protein, and are also free of gluten. More than 80% of the carb content of chia seeds is in the form of fiber. A single ounce (28 grams) of chia seeds boasts 11 grams of fiber, which is a significant portion of the reference daily intake (RDI) for women and men — 25 and 38 grams per day, respectively.

Like bananas, chia seeds contain both insoluble and soluble fiber. The fiber may also be fermented in your gut, promoting the formation of short-chain fatty acids (SCFAs) and improving colon health.

One of the unique characteristics of chia seeds is their high content of heart-healthy omega-3 fatty acids. About 75% of the fats in chia seeds consist of omega-3 alpha-linolenic acid (ALA), while about 20% consist of omega-6 fatty acids. Chia seeds are the best-known plant-based source of omega-3 fatty acids — even better than flaxseed.

Some scientists believe that a high intake of omega-3s relative to omega-6s reduces inflammation in your body.

Because they're a great source of omega-3 fatty acids, chia seeds promote a lower omega-6 to omega-3 ratio. A low ratio is associated with a lower risk of various chronic conditions — such as heart disease, cancer, and inflammatory diseases — and a lower risk of premature death.

Chia seeds contain 19% protein — a similar amount to other seeds but more than most cereals and grains. High protein intake is associated with increased fullness after meals and reduced food intake, which could contribute to weight loss.

Notably, these seeds offer all nine essential amino acids and are thus a high-quality plant-based protein, but are recommended to be part of a diet and not recommended as a stand-alone protein source.

Chia seeds provide high amounts of many minerals but not so when it comes to vitamins. Here are the minerals in chia seeds:

Manganese: Whole grains and seeds are rich in manganese, which is essential for metabolism, growth, and development

Phosphorus contributes to bone health and tissue maintenance

Copper. A mineral often lacking in the modern diet is important for heart health.

Selenium: An important antioxidant involved in many processes in your body

Iron: As a component of hemoglobin in red blood cells, iron is involved in the transport of oxygen throughout your body. It may be poorly absorbed from chia seeds due to their phytic acid content.

Magnesium plays important roles in many bodily processes

Calcium is essential for bones, muscles, and nerves

Chia seeds are very easy to incorporate into a healthy diet:

Calories: 22, Fat: 1g, Carbs: 0, Protein: 1g, Flaxseeds (1 tsp.):

The Benefits of Flaxseed

One serving of flaxseed provides a good amount of protein, fiber, and omega-3 fatty acids. It may help lower the risk of some cancers, help maintain a healthy weight, and reduce cholesterol and blood pressure.

With its mild, nutty flavor and crisp, crunchy consistency, flaxseed is a versatile ingredient that can enhance the taste and texture of almost any recipe.

One way to use this seed is by mixing it into my morning smoothie. It also makes an excellent addition to pancake batter, homemade veggie burgers, and even overnight oats. What's more, it's loaded with nutrients and linked to numerous benefits.

The benefits of flaxseed are backed by science, along with some easy ways to increase your intake. Flaxseed is one of the world's oldest crops. There are two types, brown and golden, both of which are equally nutritious. One tablespoon (7 grams) of ground flaxseed contains Calories: 37, Carbs: 2 grams, Fat: 3 grams, Fiber: 2 grams, Protein: 1.3 grams, Thiamine: 10% of the Daily Value (DV), Copper: 9% of the DV, Manganese: 8% of the DV, Magnesium: 7% of the DV, Phosphorus: 4% of the DV, Selenium: 3% of the DV, Zinc: 3% of the DV, Vitamin B6: 2% of the DV, Iron: 2% of the DV, Folate: 2% of the DV.

Flaxseed is particularly high in thiamine, a B vitamin that plays a key role in energy metabolism as well as cell function. It's also a great source of copper, which is involved in brain development, immune health, and iron metabolism.

ALA is one of the two essential fatty acids that you must obtain from the food you eat since your body doesn't produce them. Animal studies suggest that the ALA in flaxseed may help reduce inflammation and prevent cholesterol from being deposited in your heart's blood vessels.

Flaxseed is rich in lignans, which are plant compounds that have been studied for their potent cancer-fighting properties.

Interestingly, this seed boasts 75–800 times more lignans than other plant foods. Animal and test-tube studies also show flaxseed protects against colorectal, skin, blood, and lung cancer.

Also, flaxseed contains two types of fiber, — soluble and insoluble — which get fermented by the bacteria in your intestines to support gut health and improve bowel regularity. While soluble fiber absorbs water in your intestines and slows down digestion, which may help regulate blood sugar levels and lower cholesterol, insoluble fiber adds bulk to the stool, which may prevent constipation and promote regular bowel movements.

Finally, it's best to limit your intake to around 4–5 tablespoons (28–35 grams) of flaxseed per day — so you don't get too much fiber, and enjoy it as part of a healthy, balanced diet. And there you have it!

Be Blessed!

Tuna Recipe

Chickpea Tuna Salad Sandwich

Nehemiah 8:10:

"Then he said to them, "Go your way, eat the fat, drink the sweet, and send portions to those for whom nothing is prepared; for this day is holy to our Lord. Do not sorrow, for the joy of the Lord, is your strength."

This is the Soup and Sandwich Time of Year! This recipe will blow your mind! It's easy, delicious, and filling!

Ingredients:

- * 1 can (14 oz) chickpeas (garbanzo beans), drained and rinsed (Organic if possible)

- * 1 tbsp lemon juice

- * 3 – 4 tablespoons hummus (any yellow, or white)+ 2 – 3 tablespoons water;

- * 1-2 stalks of celery, chopped

- * ¼ cup red onion (about ½ small), chopped

- * 1-2 tbsp yellow or spicy mustard

- * ¼ – ½ teaspoon garlic powder

- * Celtic salt & fresh ground pepper, to taste
- Other optional ingredients: (Put Online)
- crushed nori sheets or dulse (seaweed)
- 1 tablespoon chia seeds or hemp hearts for some omega 3 & 6
- sweet or dill pickle relish
- Green and/or red peppers
- 1 tsp cayenne pepper

Health Benefits:

Chickpeas - Are a rich source of vitamins, minerals, and fiber. They aid in weight management. They make an excellent replacement for meat in many vegetarian and vegan dishes because of their texture and high protein content.

Lemon Juice - This is great for relieving sore throats. But it also has Cancer-fighting benefits, Prevents kidney stones, and aids in digestion, to name a few.

Hummus - In addition to the (chickpea) benefits above, A 2016 study explains that people who eat chickpeas or hummus eat more fiber, unsaturated fat, and vitamins and minerals than most People.

Celery - Celery is a great source of antioxidants, reduces inflammation, and supports digestion. Celery is rich in vitamins and minerals. Celery also has an alkalizing effect on the bones, helping maintain strong bone health for years to come.

Red Onions - are **rich in anthocyanins**, which are powerful plant pigments that may protect against heart disease, certain cancers, and diabetes.

Yellow Mustard - Yellow mustard can help improve the digestion of food. Studies show it can also help increase saliva production up to 8 times from consumption. And it helps accelerate the process of metabolism.

Garlic Powder - Helps the body resist or destroy viruses and other microorganisms. It does this by **boosting the immune system**.

Celtic Salt - Celtic sea salt balances out the minerals in the body and offers healing benefits. Regular consumption may help eliminate excess mucus, which in turn reduces congestion in your nasal passages and lungs.

Black Pepper - Black pepper helps to stimulate hydrochloric acid in your stomach so you can digest and absorb the foods you eat better. It has carminative properties, too, which help to reduce gas buildup in your intestines and relieve discomfort. It also helps build a strong immune system.

Seaweed - Seaweed contains many antioxidants in the form of certain vitamins (A, C, and E) and protective pigments.

It has a decent amount of iodine, a trace mineral vital for the health and function of the thyroid.

Chia Seeds - Chia seeds are healthy superfoods because they are loaded with fiber, reduce food cravings, help you stay hydrated, lower blood pressure, and are rich in omega-3 fatty acids, just to name a few.

Dill Pickle Relish - Pickles can boost your intake of antioxidants. The natural antioxidants help in the fight against free radicals. Free radicals are unstable chemicals that form naturally in the body and are linked to problems such as heart disease and cancer.

Peppers (Green/Red) - A great source of antioxidants: They contain a lot of Vitamin A, B Complex (especially Vitamin B6 and B9), and C, which can counterbalance the destructive effects of free radicals in our body and help maintain our overall health.

Leafy Greens - Some of the many benefits of eating leafy greens are reduced risk for conditions like constipation, obesity, heart disease, hypertension, and diabetes.

Cayenne Pepper - Cayenne pepper's benefits are numerous and effective; it's used to help digestion, including healing upset stomach, slowing intestinal gas, stopping stomach pain, stopping diarrhea, and as a natural remedy for cramps.

This dish is a great healthy option that will last in your fridge for several days. It's a great substitute for a cooked meal.

Instructions:

Drain and rinse the chickpeas, place in a medium-sized bowl, and roughly mash about ¾ of the chickpeas with the back of a fork or potato masher until the desired consistency is reached.

Add the rest of the ingredients and mix well, the same as making regular tuna… Add any extra ingredients you like. Alternatively, you can use a food processor to start with the beans, pulse a few times, and add the remaining ingredients, pulsing again a few times until desired consistency.

You may enjoy it chilled or at room temperature.

Ways to serve:

Ingredients To Serve With:

- 6 slices whole grain, sprouted whole grain flourless or artisan bread to serve:
  - On large leafy greens (to make a wrap)
  - Tomatoes on top
  - Spread on nori sheets,
  - With pickles,
  - *Serve as a dip for sliced vegetables

- Pair it with your favorite soup and salt-free whole-grain crackers

- Also, you may add more or less hummus to meet the desired level of moistness you want.

- (add less hummus if you like your salad on the dryer side and more if you want it moist.)

It will serve three people generously.

Store leftovers in an airtight container in the refrigerator for up to six days. Always stir before serving.

And there you have it. Enjoy!

Be Blessed!

Vegan Butternut Squash (Mac & Cheese)

Ingredients:

- 6 cups Butternut Squash (750g) Peeled and Chopped
- 11/2 Tablespoon Organic Cold Pressed Olive Oil
- 1 teaspoon Paprika
- 1/2 teaspoon Celtic Salt
- 1/2 teaspoon Crushed Black Pepper

Cashew Cheese Sauce:

- 2 cups Raw Cashews (150g)
- 4 Tablespoons Nutritional Yeast
- 1 ½ teaspoons Garlic Powder
- 1 ½ teaspoons Onion Powder
- ½ teaspoon of Oregano
- 1 teaspoon of Rosemary
- 1 ½ Tablespoon Spicy Brown Mustard
- 1 Tablespoon Lemon Juice
- 2 cups Vegetable Broth

Pasta:

- 16 ounces Chick Pea or Lentle Macaroni

Serve with freshly chopped and sprinkle with a teaspoon of:

- Basil, and or
- Parsley

Instructions:

1. Preheat the oven to 390°F (200°C).
2. Peel and cut squash into cubes, and add to a mixing bowl along with oil, garlic, paprika, salt, and pepper and toss them together well.
3. Spread it out evenly in a roasting pan or on a parchment-lined baking tray and roast in the oven for 35 minutes.
4. While the butternut squash is roasting, add raw cashews, nutritional yeast, garlic and onion powder, oregano, rosemary, mustard, lemon juice, and 1 cup of vegetable stock to the blender jug and blend until smooth. Set aside.
5. Cook and drain your pasta, before the squash finishes roasting.

6. When the butternut squash has roasted, move it to a roasting pan and add your cashew cheese sauce. Add in the remaining cup of vegetable stock and blend until you have a smooth sauce.

7. Return the cooked pasta to the pot, pour over the sauce, and gently toss it together until the pasta is well coated. Stir over low to medium heat for a few minutes to gently warm everything together.

8. Serve topped with fresh chopped parsley and basil.

Notes:

1. Place the cashews into a bowl, pour over hot water, and let them soak to soften for 15-30 minutes, then drain and rinse before blending.

2. Cook pasta according to package directions

3. You may make the sauce more nutritious by blending in more vegetables, such as broccoli, or any greens.

4. Storing and Freezing: Leftovers keep wonderfully in the fridge for 4-5 days and can be reheated in the microwave or on the stove. You can add in a dash of vegetable broth for flavor and to soften. It's also

freezer-friendly for up to 3 months if you want to freeze it.

Nutrition:

Butternut Squash - It's a good source of fiber. Foods high in dietary fiber can help keep your weight balanced and lower your cancer risk. Research shows that butternut squash can help reduce your risk of colorectal cancer, in particular. It can help your blood pressure. Butternut squash is high in potassium, which can help keep your blood pressure in check.

Olive Oil - Olive oil is also loaded with powerful antioxidants. These antioxidants are biologically active and may reduce your risk of chronic diseases. They also fight inflammation and help protect your blood cholesterol from oxidation — two benefits that may lower your risk of heart disease.

Crushed Garlic - One study found that allicin, an active component of freshly crushed garlic, had antiviral properties and was also effective against a broad range of bacteria, including multidrug-resistant strains of E. coli. It also found that allicin had antifungal properties, including against candida albicans, which causes yeast infections. It also boosts the immune system, acts as an anti-inflammatory, improves heart health, and more.

Paprika - Several paprika carotenoids, including beta carotene, lutein, and zeaxanthin, have been shown to fight oxidative stress, which is thought to increase your risk of certain cancers.

Celtic Salt - Celtic sea salt balances out the minerals in the body and offers healing benefits because it is low in sodium and high in magnesium, phosphorus, and potassium. Regular consumption may help eliminate inflammation, and excess mucus, which in turn reduces congestion in your nasal passages and lungs, to name a few benefits.

Crushed Black Pepper - Black pepper helps to stimulate hydrochloric acid in your stomach so you can digest and absorb the foods you eat better. It has carminative properties too, which help to reduce gas buildup in your intestines and relieve discomfort. It also helps build a strong immune system.

Raw Cashews - Cashews are low in sugar and rich in fiber, heart-healthy fats, and plant protein. They're also a good source of copper, magnesium, and manganese — nutrients important for energy production, brain health, immunity, and bone health. Nuts and seeds are considered antioxidant powerhouses, and cashews are no exception.

Nutritional yeast - Fortified nutritional yeast is a vegan-friendly source of protein, B vitamins, and trace minerals that support optimal health.

Garlic Powder - The most important health benefits of garlic powder include its ability to regulate high blood pressure, lower overall cholesterol levels, improve the immune system, reduce the risk of certain cancers, and aid in digestion, among others. Also, garlic powder contains vitamin C, vitamin B6, Iron, calcium, protein, magnesium, sodium, and carbohydrates, in the form of dietary fiber and sugar.

Onion Powder - Onion powder has a high content of calcium which is sufficient to keep the blood pressure regulated and promote bone health as well as support the function of the nervous system. The best benefit of onion powder is its low density of sodium. Onion powder can be replaced with salt, as it enhances the flavor of a meal.

Spicy Brown Mustard - The brown mustard seeds used to make spicy brown mustard are rich in multiple minerals, including calcium, magnesium, and potassium. A diet rich in mustard seeds can reduce inflammation and promote the healing of psoriasis-causing lesions. It is also a great antioxidant.

Lemon Juice - The health benefits of lemon juice include its ability to heal respiratory infections, treat acne, lower cholesterol, manage blood pressure levels, and detoxify the body.

Vegetable Broth - Vegetable broth is packed with minerals like calcium and magnesium and vitamins like vitamin A, C, E, and K.

Lintel Macaronie - Lentils provide a variety of health benefits and may play a role in helping people reduce or manage diabetes, obesity, cardiovascular diseases, and some cancers.

Basil - Basil contains vitamins A, and K, Calcium, Iron, and Magnesium. These nutrients and can help stave off chronic diseases, including cancer, diabetes, heart disease, and arthritis.

Parsley - Parsley works as a powerful natural diuretic and can help reduce bloating and blood pressure. Parsley is loaded with vitamin K, which has been linked to bone health. The vitamin supports bone growth and bone mineral density.

Estimated Calories: 555kcal | Carbohydrates: 87.9g | Protein: 19.1g | Fat: 14.9g | Saturated Fat: 2.5g | Sodium: 433mg | Fiber: 8.5g | Sugar: 6.4g

Be Blessed!

Rice Cakes And Avocado

Awesome Avocado and Rice Cake Snack

Ingredients:

- 2 rice cakes,
- ½ sliced avocado
- 2 Nori or other seaweed sheets (one for each rice cake
- 1 tbsp Hemp Seeds

Nutritional Information:

Brown or any flavor, rice cake - Can be a crunchy base for a delicious snack. Look for ones made with real ingredients and organic, if possible. However, the seaweed ones are also great, with that added umami punch. Opt for brown rice for a bit more fiber.

Avocado - Eating avocados helps to soothe and restore gut health, especially if you are suffering from digestive disorders such as Crohn's disease, gluten sensitivity, Celiac, colitis, or IBS. Avocados are one of the best antioxidant-rich foods and contain anti-inflammatory properties similar to that of aspirin- only without thinning the blood.

Look for ripe avocados, ones that are firm but give a little to gentle pressure.

Seaweed - Seaweed contains many antioxidants in the form of certain vitamins (A, C, and E) and protective pigments. It has a decent amount of iodine, a trace mineral vital for the health and function of the thyroid. Some seaweeds, such as purple laver, contain a good amount of B12 as well. Seaweed also has been shown to reduce cholesterol, improve gut health, reduce hunger, improve blood sugar levels, reduce the risk of cancer, and more.

Hemp seeds - Hemp Seeds are a complete protein. They have the most concentrated balance of proteins, essential fats, vitamins and enzymes combined with a relative absence of sugar, starches and saturated fats.

How to make avocado rice cakes:

1. Prep the avocado - using a knife, slice down the middle and around the avocado. Avocados have a large pit in the middle, so you won't be able to cut straight through.

Cut around the pit, then twist the avocado halves in opposite directions until they come apart. Remove the pit. You can also simply scoop out the pit with a spoon.

2. Place one sheet of seaweed on top of the rice cake, then:

3. Scoop out and slice the avocado flesh, then spread it over the seaweed. Depending on the size of the avocado, ¼ - ½ of an avocado is usually the perfect amount. Store the rest.

4. The avocado tastes like a creamy spread/dip!

5. Sprinkle the hemp seeds on top, and enjoy your delicious snack!

    Be Blessed!

Tempeh

Baked Tempeh

Prep time: five minutes; Cook time - 25 minutes; Serves 2-4 people, vegan and gluten-free.

Ingredients:

8 ounces tempeh,

1 tbsp low-sodium soy sauce (tamari), and

1 tbsp nutritional yeast

Nutritional Value Of Ingredients:

Tempeh - tempeh helps to improve digestion, reduce cholesterol, strengthen bones and improve brain function. It also boosts immunity, reduces the symptoms of PMS (pre-menstrual syndrome), fights inflammation and lowers blood pressure. You can find tempeh in multiple supermarkets today, usually tucked away in the freezer section. Also, tempeh is a great substitute for beans, as it does not cause bloating or gas.

Tamari - Tamari is a liquid condiment and popular soy sauce substitute produced through the fermentation of soybeans. Unlike regular soy sauce, little to no wheat is added during this process, resulting in a final product that is free of wheat and gluten.

Nutritional Yeast - Nutritional Yeast is high in protein, fiber and B vitamins, along with an assortment of other important vitamins and minerals. Some of the benefits include improved immunity, better digestion, and enhanced hair, skin and nail health.

Instructions:

1. Preheat the oven to 400F and line a baking sheet with parchment paper or a reusable silicone mat. Cut the tempeh into ½" cubes, then place the cubes into a small bowl.

2. Drizzle the tamari over the tempeh, then stir well. Once the tempeh has absorbed most of the liquid, sprinkle the nutritional yeast over the top and mix again. Season with any additional seasonings, if desired. Spread the tempeh out across the baking sheet, then bake on the top rack of the oven for 25-27 minutes, until golden and crispy.

(Air Fryer Option: add the tempeh to the basket of your air fryer and bake at 380F for 12-15 minutes, shaking the basket every 5 minutes.)

3. Remove from the oven and serve warm; leftovers will keep in the fridge for up to 5 days.
Enjoy!

Tofu

Baked Tofu

Baked Tofu Recipe:

Prep Time: 10 mins.

Cook Time: 30 mins.

Total Time: 40 mins.

Course: Appetizer, SideCuisine: American diet: Vegan Servings: 4 Calories: 161kcal Author: Alison Andrews.

Ingredients:

16 ounces Firm (or extra firm) Tofu (450g).

2 Tablespoons Cornstarch.

2 Tablespoons Nutritional Yeast Flakes.

1 teaspoon Garlic Powder.

1 teaspoon Onion Powder.

1/2 teaspoon Ground Ginger.

1/2 teaspoon Celtic Salt.

1/4 teaspoon Ground Black Pepper.

1/2 Tablespoon Sesame Oil.

Nutritional Value of Ingredients:

Firm Todu - Tofu is condensed soy milk that people press into blocks of different firmness. It is a nutrient-dense food that is high in protein and contains all the essential amino acids your body needs. It has also been linked to reducing heart disease, diabetes and some cancers.

Cornstarch - Cornstarch is a white, dense powder that is made from the endosperm of corn kernels. Some of the health benefits include being helpful in the management of hypoglycemia, making liquids Easier to Swallow, a healthier alternative to Corn Syrup, and making a great gluten-free alternative in Recipes.

Nutritional Yeast Flakes - Nutritional yeast is a complete protein, meaning that among the 18 amino acids it contains, nine are essential ones that your body cannot produce. Nutritional yeast also provides the compounds beta-1,3 glucan, trehalose, mannan and glutathione, which are associated with enhanced immunity, reduced cholesterol levels and cancer prevention. You get a significant dose of the minerals iron, selenium and zinc when you consume nutritional yeast as well, and one serving of nutritional yeast provides about four grams of fiber.

Garlic Powder - A February 2014 study in the Avicenna Journal of Phytomedicine reported that garlic was incorporated into treatments for many different diseases, including arthritis, respiratory infections, digestive disorders, snake and insect bites, gynecologic diseases and infectious diseases.

Garlic may also be able to help support the prevention and treatment of cardiovascular disease, reduce high blood pressure, reduce cholesterol and triglyceride levels, support the prevention and progression of cancer, reduce blood glucose levels and support the prevention of diabetes, support liver health, and support immune system function.

Garlic is also known to have beneficial antimicrobial properties and is being considered as a component of treatments for various viral, bacterial, fungal and parasitic diseases.

Onion Powder - Onions contain many antioxidants and sulfur-containing compounds. They have been linked to a reduced risk of cancer, lower blood sugar levels, and improved bone health.

Ground Ginger - Taking ginger on a daily basis can help relieve nausea, especially for pregnant women and people undergoing chemotherapy. Eating ginger could help relieve some types of pain. In particular, ginger has been found to reduce muscle soreness after exercise. Regularly consuming ginger was shown in one small study to reduce the amount of blood released during menstruation. As a result, ginger might help women who suffer from heavy periods find relief.

Celtic Salt - Humans cannot survive without salt because it helps regulate the water content in the body. Most people think they should eliminate salt from their diet, which is not a complete truth. While table salt or refined salt is toxic and unhealthy, your body needs natural pure salt to complete several processes. It means you should avoid the wrong type of salt but look for a better alternative, such as Celtic sea salt, harvested through the Celtic method that uses wooden rakes to prevent exposure to metals. The benefits of Celtic sea salt come from the way it's harvested. Celtic sea salt is sun-dried and aired in clay ponds. It is then gathered with the help of a wooden tool to ensure its living enzymes are intact. As it is unrefined salt, it provides you with 84 beneficial live elements without the addition of any preservatives or chemicals.

It's also high in sodium, an essential mineral, contains healing properties, improves cardiovascular health, promotes better brain function, alkalizes the body, stabilizes blood sugar, improves energy, prevents muscle cramps, helps kidney stones, and helps control saliva (drooling during sleep).

Black Pepper - The main active component in black pepper, piperine, is shown to decrease inflammation. Chronic inflammation can be a cause of diabetes, arthritis, asthma, and heart disease. Piperine, the active compound in black pepper, is rich in antioxidants, which prevent or delay the damaging effects of free radicals from exposure to pollution, cigarette smoke, and the sun.

Free radicals are associated with some diseases, such as heart disease and cancer. In one study, those with a diet of concentrated black pepper had less free radical damage than the group without the concentrated black pepper.

Piperine has been shown to decrease symptoms associated with Parkinson's and Alzheimer's disease, as well as improve brain function. Studies show piperine increases memory as well as the ability to decrease the production of amyloid plaques, which are damaging proteins associated with Alzheimer's disease. Pepper has been shown to improve blood sugar levels and increase the absorption of nutrients in the body.

Sesame Oil - Sesame oil is a type of vegetable oil that's made from sesame seeds.

"Sesame oil has a nutty, earthy taste to it that is very potent and aromatic. It is often used in smaller portions to cook with. Unrefined sesame oil—made by pressing roasted sesame seeds to extract their oil without refining—is also commonly used in Ayurvedic medicine.

Foods high in monounsaturated fatty acids (MUFAs), like sesame oil, have been shown to reduce cardiovascular disease risk and help manage body weight.

Polyunsaturated fatty acids (PUFAs) are another type of dietary fat found in sesame oil. They can be further broken down into omega-3 and omega-6 fatty acids. Sesame oil contains mostly omega-6 fatty acids. Omega-6 fatty acids have been shown to be beneficial for heart health and blood sugar regulation when paired with omega 3's.

Instructions:

Press your tofu, ideally using a tofu press, or place your tofu on a plate with another plate on top of it and then place something heavy on top of that, like a heavy pot or a stack of books. Let the tofu press for 30 minutes so it becomes as firm as possible.

Preheat the oven to 400°F (200°C).

Cut your pressed tofu into cubes and place it into a container with a lid.

Add the cornstarch, nutritional yeast, garlic powder, onion powder, ground ginger, salt, and ground black pepper to a bowl and mix together.

Drizzle the sesame oil over the tofu, and then put the lid on the container and rotate it a few times so that the oil is evenly spread.

Add the cornstarch and seasonings mix to the tofu, and then put the lid on again and rotate the bowl a few times so that the tofu is evenly coated with the spices.

Spread the tofu cubes evenly on a parchment-lined baking tray.

Bake for 15 minutes and then flip the tofu cubes and bake for a further 15 minutes until deliciously crispy.

Notes

Tofu: If your tofu is super extra firm, then you may be able to skip the step of pressing it first. However, the issue is that if you think your tofu is super firm, but it isn't really, then when you rotate it in the bowl with the spices, it will break up. A tofu press is highly recommended if you eat tofu regularly.

Serving: This is totally delicious and served with some sweet chili sauce or vegan BBQ sauce for dipping or a vegan peanut sauce.

Prep Time: This does not include the time taken to press the tofu.

This recipe will provide a great high-protein meal and should come out super crispy and tasty.

Nutrition

Serving: 1Serve | Calories: 161kcal | Carbohydrates: 6.4g | Protein: 14.4g | Fat: 8.5g | Saturated Fat: 1.5g | Sodium: 409mg | Fiber: 0.4g | Sugar: 0.9g.

Be Blessed!

Seitan

Seitan Fajita Bowl:

Servings: 4, Prep Time: 10 min., Cook Time: 20 min., Total Time: 30 minutes.

*People with certain health conditions—specifically, those with a wheat allergy, celiac disease, or non-celiac gluten sensitivity-should avoid Seitan because the main ingredient is wheat.

Ingredients

2 cups cooked quinoa

2 tablespoons olive oil

5 cloves garlic, *minced*

1 large red bell pepper, *or any colour you desire, sliced*

1 package seitan, *12 ounces, sliced*

1 cup baby bella mushrooms, *sliced*

1/2 cup cherry tomatoes, *sliced*

1/2 teaspoon cumin

1/2 teaspoon chili powder

1/4 teaspoon red pepper flakes

1/4 teaspoon oregano

1/4 teaspoon onion powder

salt and pepper to taste

2 cups canned black beans, *drained*

2 cups lettuce, *shredded*

Nutritional Value of Ingredients:

Quinoa - Quinoa is a highly nutritious plant that is grown as a crop because of its edible seeds. Compared to many grains, the seeds of the quinoa plant have more nutritional value in protein, dietary fiber, and B vitamins. It is also an excellent source of carbohydrates, protein, and fats. Studies have shown that eating this food daily can reduce risks of cancer, cardiovascular diseases, high blood sugar, and respiratory tract problems by up to seventeen percent.

Olive Oil - Olive oil may offer health benefits as it is high in healthy monosaturated fats and antioxidants. Olive oil has a host of health benefits, including anti-inflammatory properties. It also helps in preventing stroke, protects against heart disease, may fight against Alzheimer's disease, reduces the risk of type II diabetes, has anti-cancer properties, helps treat rheumatoid arthritis, and has anti-bacterial properties.

Garlic - Garlic (such as garlic extract or powder) could be a helpful side therapy for those already being treated for cardiovascular disease, high blood pressure, **and diabetes**, and potentially may even reduce the risk of heart attack and stroke.

Another study published in 2017 involving an analysis of nine clinical trials with a total of 768 patients with type 2 diabetes found that those who took 50 to 1,500 mg of a garlic supplement each day for two or three months had significant reductions in their fasting blood glucose levels.

In an earlier, smaller study of 55 people with metabolic syndrome—a group of risk factors, such as excess stomach fat or high blood pressure, that raise the risk of heart disease—published in the Journal of Nutrition, Budoff and his colleagues found that those who took a daily garlic supplement for a year had slower plaque buildup from coronary artery disease than those who took a placebo.

Bell Pepper -One of the benefits of bell peppers is the high presence of vitamin B6, which increases the levels of serotonin and norepinephrine, sometimes referred to as the "happy hormones."

Seitan - Seitan (pronounced say-tan) is a good source of plant-based protein that is made from wheat gluten. It is extremely versatile in the kitchen. Seitan is especially useful for those who, for whatever reason, cannot eat soy protein.

Mushrooms - Mushrooms lower pressure, help to boost the immune system and are a rich, low-calorie source of fiber, protein and antioxidants. They may also mitigate the risk of developing serious health conditions, such as Alzheimer's, heart disease, cancer and diabetes.

Cherry Tomatoes - Cherry tomatoes are low in calories but high in fibre, vitamins A and C, and carotenoid antioxidants such as lutein, lycopene, and beta-carotene. Studies show cherry tomatoes may protect heart health, lower your risk of certain diseases, and support healthy skin by protecting against the harmful effects of UV light.

Cumin - Modern research shows cumin promotes better digestion by increasing the digestive enzymes, potentially speeding up digestion. Cumin is also a rich source of iron and contains lots of plant compounds that are linked with potential health benefits, including terpenes, phenols, flavonoids and alkaloids. Last but not least, cumin has antimicrobial properties that may reduce the risk of food-borne infections.

Chili Powder - Some health benefits of chili powder include improving your eyesight and preventing night blindness and macular degeneration from developing as we age. Chili powder contains copper and iron, which contribute to the formation of new blood cells, which will prevent anemia, fatigue, and muscular weakness. Chili powder also improves cognitive function, helps maintain healthy blood pressure, And it contains vitamin C, a potent natural water-soluble antioxidant that helps the body develop resistance against infectious agents and eliminates cancer-causing free radicals in the body.

Red Pepper Flakes - Red bell pepper contains beta-cryptoxanthin, a compound that your body turns into vitamin A. Research suggests foods rich in beta-cryptoxanthin may help lower the risk of bladder, lung and colon cancer.

Oregano -

Oregano is rich in antioxidants; Oregano is rich in antioxidants, which are compounds that help fight damage from harmful free radicals in the body. It may help fight bacteria, cancer, and reduce viral infections, decrease inflammation.

Onion Powder - Onions contain many antioxidants and sulfur-containing compounds. They have been linked to a reduced risk of cancer, lower blood sugar levels, and improved bone health.

Salt/Pepper - Humans cannot survive without salt because it helps regulate the water content in the body. Most people think they should eliminate salt from their diet, which is not a complete truth. While table salt or refined salt is toxic and unhealthy, your body needs natural pure salt to complete several processes. It means you should avoid the wrong type of salt but look for a better alternative, such as Celtic sea salt, harvested through the Celtic method that uses wooden rakes to prevent exposure to metals. The benefits of Celtic sea salt come from the way it's harvested. Celtic sea salt is sun-dried and aired in clay ponds. It is then gathered with the help of a wooden tool to ensure its living enzymes are intact. As it is unrefined salt, it provides you with 84 beneficial live elements without the addition of any preservatives or chemicals.

It's also high in sodium, an essential mineral, contains healing properties, improves cardiovascular health, promotes better brain function, alkalizes the body, stabilizes blood sugar, improves energy, prevents muscle cramps, helps kidney stones, and helps control saliva (drooling while sleeping).

The main active component in black pepper, piperine, is shown to decrease inflammation.[4] Chronic inflammation can be a cause of diabetes, arthritis, asthma, and heart disease. Piperine, the active compound in black pepper, is rich in antioxidants, which prevent or delay the damaging effects of free radicals from exposure to pollution, cigarette smoke, and the sun.

Free radicals are associated with some diseases, such as heart disease and cancer. In one study, those with a diet of concentrated black pepper had less free radical damage than the group without the concentrated black pepper.

Piperine has been shown to decrease symptoms associated with Parkinson's and Alzheimer's disease, as well as improve brain function.[7] Studies show piperine increased memory as well as the ability to decrease the production of amyloid plaques, which are damaging proteins associated with Alzheimer's disease. Pepper has been shown to improve blood sugar levels and increase the absorption of nutrients in the body.

Lettuce - Lettuce is an excellent source of fiber and cellulose, which improves digestion and promotes long-term weight loss. It is also rich in vitamin A, vitamin C, vitamin E, and vitamin K, as well as minerals including potassium, magnesium, iron, calcium, and zinc.

Black Beans - There are so many benefits to eating black beans. Calcium is great for strong bones; however, black beans are rich in minerals like magnesium, iron, zinc, calcium, phosphorous, manganese and copper, which are essential for strong bones and building a strong bone structure. And they contribute to reducing all metabolic diseases.

Per Bowl Instructions:

1/2 cup quinoa

1 cup lettuce, *shredded*

1/2 cup Black Beans

1/4 cup sautéed red bell peppers

sautéed tomatoes

sautéed mushrooms

1/4 serving cooked seitan

lime wedges *to serve and squeeze over*

Vegan Fajita Bowl Instructions:

Cook the quinoa according to package directions and mix in 2 teaspoons maple syrup and lime. See here how to cook quinoa:

While the quinoa is cooking, heat the olive oil in a large pan over medium-high heat.

Add the minced garlic and sauté until fragrant. Add in the sliced bell peppers, the seitan slices, mushrooms and tomatoes. Stir together, add all the seasonings and stir in. Reduce heat to medium and allow all the ingredients to cook until softened, for about 15 minutes. Add in the black beans to heat through and mix in with the rest of the ingredients. Add salt and pepper to taste, and add more seasonings if desired.

Remove from heat.

Per bowl, add ½ cup quinoa ¼ cup lettuce and split the rest of the ingredients into four equal bowls in desired quantities. Serve with lime wedges on the side, and enjoy!

Be Blessed!

Black Beans

How to Cook Black Beans:

Prep Time: 10 mins, Cook Time: 1 hr 20 mins, Serves 12

Ingredients:

2 cups dried black beans

8 cups water, more as needed

2 teaspoons cumin

1 teaspoon (Optional: extra-virgin olive oil)

2 teaspoons sea salt

Freshly ground black pepper

1 (3-inch) piece of kombu, rinsed, optional (see note)

3 garlic cloves, grated

Optional add-ins:

Chili powder

Mexican oregano

Lime juice and zest

Chopped cilantro

Instructions:

Place the beans in a large colander and sort through them to remove and discard any stones or debris.

Rinse the beans and transfer them to a large pot or Dutch oven. Add the water, cumin, olive oil, salt, and pepper, and bring to a boil. Reduce the heat, add the kombu, if using, and simmer, uncovered, until the beans are tender. I like to check mine starting at 1 hour and every 15 minutes after that. Depending on the freshness of your beans, it could take up to 2½ hours. Add more liquid to the pot, as needed, to keep your beans submerged.

Remove the kombu and add the garlic during the last few minutes of cooking.

Season the beans as you like, adding chili powder, oregano, and more salt and pepper, if desired. Let the beans cool in the cooking liquid (I like how it gets nice and thick). Just before serving, stir in lime juice, zest, and cilantro, if desired.

Nutritional Value of Ingredients:

Dried Black Beans - Black beans are heart-friendly and anticancer. Black beans contain plant compounds called flavonoids, which have powerful anti-inflammatory properties. Reducing inflammation is key in protecting yourself from heart disease and every type of cancer. Black beans are also rich in soluble fiber.

Cumin - Cumin aids digestion by increasing the activity of digestive proteins. It may also reduce symptoms of irritable bowel syndrome. Cumin is very dense in iron, providing almost 20% of your daily iron in one teaspoon. Free radicals are lone electrons that cause inflammation and damage DNA. Cumin contains antioxidants that stabilize free radicals. Cumin supplements have improved blood cholesterol in multiple studies. It is unclear if using cumin in small amounts as a seasoning has the same benefits. Cumin extracts reduce signs of narcotic addiction in mice. It is not yet known if they would have similar effects in humans. Cumin contains multiple plant compounds that decrease inflammation in test-tube studies.

Extra Virgin Olive Oil - The biggest thing that makes extra virgin olive oil so healthy is its unique disease-fighting component, polyphenols. Polyphenols are a potent antioxidant.

Sea Salt - Humans cannot survive without salt because it helps regulate the water content in the body. Most people think they should eliminate salt from their diet, which is not a complete truth. While table salt or refined salt is toxic and unhealthy, your body needs natural pure salt to complete several processes. It means you should avoid the wrong type of salt but look for a better alternative such as Celtic sea salt, harvested through the Celtic method that uses wooden rakes to prevent exposure to metals. The benefits of Celtic sea salt come from the way it's harvested. Celtic sea salt is sun-dried and aired in clay ponds. It is then gathered with the help of a wooden tool to ensure its living enzymes are intact. As it is unrefined salt, it provides you with 84 beneficial live elements without the addition of any preservatives or chemicals.

It's also high in sodium, an essential mineral, contains healing properties, improves cardiovascular health, promotes better brain function, alkalizes the body, stabilizes blood sugar, improves energy, prevents muscle cramps, helps kidney stones, and helps control saliva (drooling while sleeping).

Ground Black Pepper - The main active component in black pepper, piperine, is shown to decrease inflammation.[4] Chronic inflammation can be a cause of diabetes, arthritis, asthma, and heart disease. Piperine, the active compound in black pepper, is rich in antioxidants, which prevent or delay the damaging effects of free radicals from exposure to pollution, cigarette smoke, and the sun.

Free radicals are associated with some diseases, such as heart disease and cancer. In one study, those with a diet of concentrated black pepper had less free radical damage than the group without the concentrated black pepper.

Piperine has been shown to decrease symptoms associated with Parkinson's and Alzheimer's disease, as well as improve brain function.[7] Studies show piperine increased memory as well as the ability to decrease the production of amyloid plaques, which are damaging proteins associated with Alzheimer's disease. Pepper has been shown to improve blood sugar levels and increase the absorption of nutrients in the body.

Kombu - Researchers know that seaweed can provide a relatively inexpensive and environmentally-friendly combination of high-quality protein, healthy fats, fiber, and other nutrients.

Garlic Cloves - Raw garlic has anti-inflammatory, antioxidative, antibacterial, and anticancer properties.

Notes:

Store the beans in an airtight container in the fridge for up to five days or freeze them for several months. The beans can be stored in the cooking liquid or drained and stored.

The kombu is optional, but it helps the beans become more digestible. Kombu can get bitter if boiled, so be sure to keep your beans cooking at a gentle simmer after you add it.

Enjoy!

Be Blessed!

Salad

Tossed Green Salad

The following ingredients are some of the healthiest ones you can include in a salad:

Red Or Green Leaf Lettuce - Both are rich in vitamins A and K; the green leaf is higher in vitamin C. Red leaf lettuce gets its color from the flavonoid antioxidant anthocyanin, which may help lower levels of LDL (bad) cholesterol.

Carrots - Eating carrots is linked to a reduced risk of cancer and heart disease, as well as improved eye health. Additionally, this vegetable may be a valuable component of an effective weight loss diet.

Yellow Peppers - Like other fruits and vegetables, bell peppers may have many health benefits. These include improved eye health and reduced risk of anemia.

Spinach - Spinach boasts many plant compounds that can improve health, such as lutein, kaempferol, nitrates, quercetin, and zeaxanthin. Spinach is extremely healthy and linked to numerous health benefits. It has been shown to improve oxidative stress, eye health, and blood pressure. Free radicals are byproducts of metabolism.

Broccoli - Broccoli supports a healthy immune system by supplying the body with vitamin C and sulforaphanes. Sulforaphanes stimulate an immune response to kick-start the antioxidant and anti-inflammatory responses within the body. This mechanism is crucial to ensure infection-causing bacteria cannot survive within cells.

Beans And Legumes - Black beans are heart-friendly and anticancer. Black beans contain plant compounds called flavonoids, which have powerful anti-inflammatory properties. Reducing inflammation is key in protecting yourself from heart disease and every type of cancer. Black beans are also rich in soluble fiber.

Studies show that legumes can guard against type-2 diabetes, Improve glycemic and lipid control for people who have diabetes, lower blood pressure and cholesterol, help control weight and lower your risk of heart disease.

Olive Oil - Olive oil may offer health benefits as it is high in healthy monosaturated fats and antioxidants. Olive oil has a host of health benefits, including anti-inflammatory properties. It also helps in preventing stroke, protects against heart disease, may fight against Alzheimer's disease, reduces the risk of type II diabetes, has anti-cancer properties, helps treat rheumatoid arthritis, and has anti-bacterial properties.

Balsamic Vinegar - It helps lower cholesterol. It aids in healthy digestion. It supports weight loss. It's diabetes-friendly, It improves blood circulation, It may help with hypertension. It can improve your skin.

Sunflower Seeds - Sunflower seeds are incredibly good for you. They have a number of health benefits. For example, they can aid in reducing inflammation. By consuming them five or more times a week, a study showed that they lowered inflammation levels. In addition, sunflower seeds, being rich in healthy fats, help with heart health, reducing cardiovascular diseases and reducing the risks of strokes and heart failures. Sunflower seeds also boost the immune system through their supply of zinc and selenium, vital minerals that aid in developing white blood cells and boosting immunity. They also boost energy levels due to the presence of vitamin B1, which helps with digestion and thus helps you keep up your energy throughout the day.

Flaxseeds - Flaxseed is an important addition to many diets, offering health benefits for everything from heart health to blood sugar levels.

The vitamins, minerals, and fiber in flaxseed can provide important health benefits. Magnesium, for example, is important for more than 300 different reactions in your body.

Magnesium is also important for strong bones and helps build your DNA.

Flaxseed also provides a significant amount of choline, which helps your body's cells communicate with each other.

Compounds called lignans have been linked to a lower risk of cancer, especially prostate and breast cancer. Flaxseed is one of the best natural sources of lignans, containing as much as 800 times more than other plants.

Flaxseed is often used as a fiber supplement because of the large amounts of dietary fiber it contains. Flaxseed has both insoluble and soluble forms of dietary fiber, which can improve your digestive system in several ways. Insoluble fiber adds bulk to your stool, helping your intestines process waste more effectively. Soluble fiber turns into a type of gel in your stomach and helps absorb cholesterol before it ever makes it to your bloodstream.

Tomatoes - Tomatoes help to keep your digestive system healthy by keeping both constipation and diarrhea at bay. Also, it effectively prevents jaundice and removes harmful toxins from your body. Moreover, a large amount of fiber in tomatoes may bulk up the stool and relieve the symptoms of constipation.

Almonds - Antioxidants in almonds have been shown to reduce blood pressure. Increasing the level of magnesium through the oral dietary intake of almonds may contribute to maintaining healthy blood pressure. Almonds have been found to reduce 'bad' cholesterol in the blood while supporting the maintenance of 'good' cholesterol.

Cauliflower - Cauliflower is a good source of fibre and vitamins. It's known to strengthen bones, boost the cardiovascular system, and prevent cancer. If using blood thinners, you should consult with your doctor before eating cauliflower, as it contains high levels of vitamin K, which could react adversely with the drugs.

Garlic - Garlic and garlic supplements may help prevent and reduce the severity of illnesses like the flu and the common cold. Garlic contains antioxidants that can help protect against cognitive decline related to cell damage and aging. This may reduce your risk (or slow the progression) of Alzheimer's disease and other types of dementia.

Brussels Sprouts - Brussels sprouts are low in calories, but high in many nutrients, especially fiber, vitamin K, and vitamin C. Brussels sprouts are high in antioxidants. This helps prevent cell damage in your body. Brussels sprouts are high in fiber, which can promote regularity, support digestive health, and reduce the risk of heart disease and diabetes. Brussels sprouts are high in vitamin K, a nutrient important for blood clotting and bone metabolism.

Kale - Many powerful antioxidants are found in kale, including quercetin and kaempferol, which have numerous beneficial effects on health. Kale contains substances that bind bile acids and lower cholesterol levels in the body. Steamed kale is particularly effective. As a nutrient-dense, low-calorie food, kale makes an excellent addition to a weight-loss diet.

Green Peas - Green peas are a great source of many carotenoid vitamin A-like compounds, which help preserve eye function and buffer oxidative damage to the sensitive structures within.

Swiss Chard - Chard contains three times the recommended daily intake of vitamin K and 44 percent of the recommended amount of vitamin A. The vegetable can help to combat cancer, reduce blood pressure, and enhance performance in sports.

Collard Greens - Collard greens are nutrient-dense and low in calories. They're an excellent source of calcium, folate, and vitamins K, C, and A. Furthermore, they're high in fiber and antioxidants.

Collard greens may protect against cancer and improve bone, eye, digestive, and heart health.

Ingredients:

5 cups loosely packed mixed greens - or any favorite lettuce

2 tablespoons shelled sunflower seeds

¼ red onion - thinly sliced

1 cucumber - peeled and thinly sliced

2 stalks of celery - chopped

Bonus - light vinaigrette dressing recipe:

¼ cup Dijon mustard

¼ cup honey

¼ cup apple cider vinegar

1 teaspoon salt

¼ teaspoon black pepper

¼ cup oil - I use extra virgin olive oil

And any of the above ingredients you desire

Instructions:

Combine dressing ingredients in a jar, cover, and shake vigorously to combine.

In a large bowl, combine mixed greens, sunflower seeds, bacon, red onions, and cucumbers. Just before serving, add dressing to taste and toss to combine. Serve immediately after tossing with dressing.

Enjoy!

Nutrition:

Approximate Calories: 179 kcal, Carbohydrates: 15 g, Protein: 4 g, Fat: 13 g, Saturated Fat: 2 g, Trans Fat: 1 g, Cholesterol: 7 mg, Sodium: 661 mg, Potassium: 135 mg, Fiber: 1 g, Sugar: 13 g, Vitamin A: 54 IU, Vitamin C: 2 mg, Calcium: 19 mg, Iron: 1 mg;

Be Blessed!

Acknowledgments

I want to thank my handsome husband, James Roberts, for always supporting me in my endeavors, from going back to school in my 40s to competing in bodybuilding, writing this book, and everything in between. James is a former NC State Champion bodybuilder, retired military, and technical engineer. He is currently working in the field of lifestyle and wellness coaching. He is a personal trainer, holistic nutritionist, and motivational speaker as well. Over the years, we have worked together on a number of projects, including good fellowship conferences, NC A&T State University's alumni fitness programs, health awareness programs including Live Life, Lupus event, Esteem, A Total Transformation, A Non-Profit Holistic Health Organization and co-producer of Living Fit With James And Karen Roberts, on 100.7 FM Radio Greensboro, NC.

I love you, and thank you for being an awesome, patient, and loving husband!

I also want to thank one of the most amazing people I know, the beautiful Dr. Dianne (Dee)Wellington. Dianne, a client of mine for many years, also became a great friend and was a Ph.D. Grad Student at the onset of this project. She has achieved a second master's degree and a Ph.D. She is an avid researcher and university professor (currently at SUNY Cortland and NCA&T State University) and has published multiple literature papers in her own right. She is a highly sought-after international speaker, researcher, and educator in diversity. Dianne is not just brains and beauty; even though we are currently in two different locations, she still works out most days, sometimes twice a day, and follows a healthy eating regimen. Dianne has a close relationship with her friends and family, making it her mission to spend quality time with them as often as possible. And with all that on her plate, she still manages to coach me with every aspect of this book, from cover to cover. I love you, and thank you for your love and support!

And finally, I would also like to thank my friends, family, and clients for their love and support over the years (too many to list.). Many of whom I worked with over the years. It has been through these relationships that I developed the desire to share this information with the hope of helping others live a better, healthier, more productive lifestyle, that they can then share with their family, friends, and on and on.

Finally, I would like to thank my family, friends, church, and radio family, including Bishop Michael Thomas, Linda Greenwood of Love, Faith Christian Fellowship, and the 100.7 FM The Joy Radio Program. Many of whom I worked with over the years. Through these relationships, I developed the desire to share this information with the hope of helping others live a better, healthier, more productive lifestyle that they can then share with their family, friends, and so on. Much love!

About The Author

Karen Roberts is a resident of Greensboro, NC, a North Carolina A&T State University Aggie, and a Graduate of The University of North Carolina at Greensboro, a Certified Personal Trainer, Certified Sports Nutritionist, and Certified Forks over Knives Instructor. Karen is also a competitive bodybuilder, competition judge, and trainer. She has been in the fitness industry for over 40 years.

As a wellness coach and personal trainer, Karen has had the opportunity to guide clients to living a healthier lifestyle; this lifestyle includes the spiritual, physical, mental, and social aspects of life. She teaches the importance of taking time for spiritual acknowledgment, eating healthy, getting rest, working out, and having an active social life, whether it be going to the movies or spending time with friends and family.

Karen has helped countless clients lose weight (upwards of 100 pounds in some cases), come off their medications, lose 10, 20, and 30% or more of body fat, and dramatically change the direction of their lives. For Karen, the goal is to live until you die and to understand the body is self-healing. Thus, if you live healthily, there will be little to no need for medications, procedures, or surgeries.

Karen is a motivational speaker, engaging in events from churches, to non-profit wellness organizations. She has had the honor of being a guest on Spectrum News (Raleigh, NC), as a fitness advisor.

For the past seven years, Karen has co-hosted with her husband, James Roberts, "Living Fit with James and Karen Roberts." A radio program [100.7 FM The Joy WLJF; (https://streema.com/radios/WLJF_LP)] that coaches a health and wellness lifestyle using spiritual principles from the Bible. This program, is what inspired Karen to write this book. Karen wants to share the natural benefits of wellness with people of all backgrounds, regardless of their religion, race, age, and sex.

When not working, Karen enjoys traveling, going to the beach, and spending time with her friends and family, especially her husband, James, and her four grown sons, two daughters-in-law, and three grandchildren. She also weight trains five to six days a week, goes for hikes, loves to bike ride, and cooks vegan dishes from scratch. In general, Karen is very motivated to help others live a healthier lifestyle, and she hopes this book will be an attribute to that.